Ask the Doctor
Hypertension

Ask the Doctor
Hypertension

By Vince Friedewald, M.D.

Andrews and McMeel

A Universal Press Syndicate Company

Kansas City

Library of Congress Cataloging-in-Publication Data

Friedewald, Vincent E., 1941–
    Ask the doctor : hypertension / by Vince
Friedewald.
            p.   cm.
    Includes bibliographical references and index.
    ISBN 0–8362–7022–3
    1. Hypertension—Popular works. I. Title.
RC685.H8F73   1995
616.´32—dc20
94–46904

CIP

In memory of my parents,
Eleanor and Vincent Friedewald

Contents

Acknowledgments

WHEN MY DAD realized how much I loved to write, he told me that if I became a physician, I would have plenty to write about.

As usual, Pop was right. Consequently, *Ask the Doctor: Hypertension* is only the first of a whole series of books dedicated to his life's devotion: helping folks who are ill. That's what he did better than any other doctor I've ever known. Just ask any of the thousands of his patients across the desolate plains of West Texas, and they'll tell you what I mean.

Now you know where the inspiration for *Ask the Doctor* comes from.

But it takes more than inspiration to create such books. That's where thousands of people—researchers and clinicians, doctors and nurses, hospital technicians and pharmaceutical company scientists, and patients themselves—play an essential role. Every word in *Ask the Doctor* is the result of their contributions to the vast wealth of information about hypertension.

And where do you find this information? Here are some of our sources: *American Journal of Cardiology, American Heart Journal, American Journal of Medicine, Annals of Internal Medicine, Archives of Internal Medicine, British Medical Journal, Circulation, Consultant, Contemporary Medicine, Drug Therapy, Hospital Medicine, JNC V, Journal Watch, JAMA, Journal of the American College of Cardiology, Lancet, Merck Manual, Modern Medicine, New England Journal of Medicine, Patient Care, Physician's Desk Reference,* and *Scientific American Medicine.*

And who were the authors of these publications? The answer is borrowed from the standard medical laboratory abbreviation "TNTC," or "Too numerous to count." Let's just say, you know who you are, and thank you for making *Ask the Doctor* possible.

I also wish to thank Chris Crossen for his outstanding editorial contributions throughout the development of the book; Tony Edens for encouraging me to pursue the project; my terrific staff at American Medical Communications; and the wonderful people at the University of Notre Dame, especially Dan Crossen in the Development Office and Mary Mitchell in the Department of Communication and Theater.

I am also delighted to recognize the contribution of John McMeel, who had the courage to trust a doctor to write a book after listening to the *Ask the Doctor* idea at a football game, as well as the generous help of John's great team at Andrews and McMeel.

Finally, special gratitude to my wife, Julie, for the love and support she always provides regardless of how crazy my newest venture may seem; and to Natalie and Vincent, the two best kids a father could ever lay claim to, for making it all worthwhile.

And sorry, everybody. This is just the beginning.

Introducing:
A New Journey

Two snakes met on a garden path. One snake was
coughing, his eyes bulging.

"You look awful," said the other snake.

"I just had a terrible experience at my doctor's office,"
replied the first snake.

"What happened?"

"They took my blood pressure."

"That's wonderful. Everyone should have their blood
pressure checked," the second snake said.

"You wouldn't think so if someone pumped up a cuff
around *your* neck."

IF YOU HAVE HIGH blood pressure, consider yourself lucky you're
not a snake.

You're lucky for another reason. You found this book—or
maybe this book found you. Either way, we're taking you on a
journey like you've never taken before.

Journey?

Yes, a journey. That's why *Ask the Doctor* looks more like a travel
guide than another (yawn) medical book.

Controlling high blood pressure, you see, is like a journey to a
foreign land. . . .

- The most important thing is to make the trip safely.

- A little advance knowledge about where you're going
  makes the trip a lot better.

- It's a new experience, filled with all sorts of unknowns.

- There are some strange words you should learn to get along.

- The food may be different.

- It can be expensive, but there are ways to save money.

- There are lots of misconceptions about this strange land.

- A good sense of humor helps a lot.

- Your travel agent (your doctor) will make all the arrangements, but it's up to you to make the journey.

So how do you use *Ask the Doctor*?

Just like a travel guide. First you read it, cover to cover. You'll learn lots of valuable information, like details of the hotel you'll stay in. But there's a lot you won't remember until you are actually there, such as the many small towns you'll be traveling through. That's when you will want to read some more. So you take the guide with you on your trip.

Same thing with *Ask the Doctor*. There's a great deal you'll find out your first time through the book. But you shouldn't even try to remember the details of the hundreds of medications your doctor can choose from after one read. When your doctor prescribes that little pill to take every morning, you'll already have a good general idea about antihypertensive medications. Then you can reopen the book and read in more detail about your treatment.

To help you return to *Ask the Doctor* for specific questions about medications, exercise, diet, and many other things that are going to cross your mind, we've designed special icons to help you find things more easily. Be sure to get aquainted with them—they're an easy way to find things quickly.

Here's another tip. We don't want you to just read *Ask the Doctor*. Since you are actually taking the journey, we've put a section called "It's Your Turn" at the end of each chapter. These are questions for *you*. If you don't know the answers, you should find out.

Maybe the story about the snakes didn't make you roll on the floor in laughter (if it did, you may have another problem). But hypertension is a serious problem, and we don't think that a smile now and then is such a bad idea. Laughter may not really be the *best* medicine, but it sure can help.

How about language? We're not bashful about using medical terms. Doctors use them for good reason—no, not to hide from you what they're talking about, but because certain words describe exactly what we're talking about. It's important that you learn some of these words yourself. After all, they are about *your* health. These words are identified in the book margin by the doctor icon.

Finally, a word about accuracy. Everything we have to say is based on what the experts generally agree on, based on their writings and a document called the *Joint National Committee on Detection, Evaluation, and Treatment of High Blood Pressure*. We'll just refer to it as *JNC V*. But, as you are soon to find out, there's a lot to say about hypertension, far more than we could pack into *Ask the Doctor*. So just because we don't mention something between these two covers doesn't necessarily mean it isn't true, or not important.

Furthermore, things change. The day after these pages are printed, we could learn something different about almost *anything* we said. Another problem is that experts don't always agree with each other, and your doctor may not necessarily agree with the experts. All of which is to say that somebody, somewhere, may not agree with us, either.

So what do you do? *Ask the Doctor* may be the best book ever written on hypertension, but it's still just a book, not your doctor. Never do anything based solely on what we say. Instead, the final word in all matters related to your hypertension is your personal physician. In other words, ASK THE REAL DOCTOR, *your* doctor, before you change or make any new plans in your journey with hypertension.

Bon voyage!

Icons

Throughout *Ask the Doctor*, you will see a number of icons, symbols in the margins of each page, used to emphasize important specific information. We have arranged the icons in such a way that it is very easy to use them as reference guides. For example, if you want to read all about sodium in relation to hypertension, you could page through *Ask the Doctor* and look for all the paragraphs with the saltshaker icon. The same goes for age-related topics, lifestyle changes, and information on target organ disease.

The icons complement the index in the back of the book. In fact, they're just a very quick reference guide to help you look up any information you may want to get to quickly.

 "doctorspeak," medical definitions and terminology

 age-related topics, both elderly and young

 very important information you should pay special attention to

 alcohol-related topics

 diet-related topics

 gender-specific information

 salt- and sodium-related topics

 exercise, lifestyle changes

 blood pressure-specific information: numbers, stages, etc.

 target organ disease

 race-related topics

 "It's Your Turn" sections at the end of each chapter

 weight-related topics

 family, heredity

 medication/drug information and topics

 cost

 stress-related topics

 tobacco

1

What Is Hypertension?

ONE SUNNY DAY three or four hundred million years ago, give or take a few million years, a very small ocean creature was caught in a breaking wave and washed up on an uninhabited beach. It was uninhabited because, at that time in the history of our planet, all the creatures lived in the sea.

Our little friend gazed up and down the deserted beach, and liked what it saw. But as much as it wanted to stay, it couldn't. That's because its tissues needed to get their oxygen and food directly from the sea. Unable to remain, it rode the next wave back out to sea.

Apparently the Lord was watching that day and it occurred to him that maybe there ought to be creatures on the land as well as the oceans of the wonderful planet He had created. Problem was, how could they get that food and oxygen to the various parts of their bodies?

Of course the Lord isn't ever stumped by anything for very long. He figured all the creatures that needed to live on land would have a network of small tubes, *blood vessels*, through which salt water could travel to all parts of their little bodies. Which meant that there'd have to be *pressure* inside the vessels, to make the water flow forward. So he designed a special pump, the *heart*, to generate the right amount of pressure.

And it wasn't too many million years later when lots of creatures, big and small, were roaming the earth, each constantly fed by circulating fluids very similar to the waters of the sea. A few more million years went by, and a creature that never lived in the sea, a human, began walking the earth. Humans, too, were sustained by salt water, under *pressure*, in the form of *blood*.

A true story, more or less.

SO BLOOD PRESSURE is a good thing. It lets us live outside the ocean, for starters. But good things can go bad, like when people get hypertension.

Hypertension is a disease in which the blood pressure is elevated most of the time, day and night, during rest and activity, eating and sleeping, work and play. Hypertension is also a *risk factor* for other diseases; if left untreated, it leads to damage of the heart, kidneys, brain, and the blood vessels themselves.

Over sixty million people have hypertension, which afflicts persons of all ages, both sexes, and all ethnic backgrounds. It may occur in a single family member, but runs in families, too. High blood pressure is often present along with other diseases, such as diabetes mellitus, that also tend to occur in blood relatives.

Doctors classify hypertension into two types: *primary* hypertension (over 90% of people with hypertension have this form) and *secondary* hypertension, which means that the blood pressure is elevated due to the presence of another disease, most often involving the kidneys.

But before we can really understand hypertension, we must first understand just what blood pressure itself is. Then we'll come back to hypertension.

> **Risk Factor:** Something that increases the chances for a disease or other form of ill health to occur.

What Is Blood Pressure?

Turn on your water faucet. Ever think about how the water gets there? The answer is *pressure*. By applying pressure generated by pumps, water constantly flows forward from the city's reservoirs, into the water mains, and finally into the pipes in your home.

The same is true in your body, whose every cell needs blood to survive. Your heart is the pump that creates the pressure inside the blood vessels, pushing blood into the vast network of blood vessels from the surface of your scalp to the tips of your toes.

Let's learn more about how this works, because your understanding of blood pressure is key to how you are going to control high blood pressure.

Doctors call your blood vessels and heart the *cardiovascular system*. That's what we're going to call it, too.

The heart of the cardiovascular system is the heart. The heart has only one purpose: to pump blood. It does this by keeping the pressure high enough so that every part of the body always receives enough blood to carry out its job. This may be the leg muscles climbing stairs, the stomach and intestines digesting food, or the uterus supplying sugar and oxygen to a baby in the womb.

Cardio = **Heart**
Vascular = **Blood Vessel**
Your cardiovascular system is made up of the heart and three types of blood vessels: arteries, veins, and capillaries. When we refer to the BP, we are concerned only with the pressure inside the arteries.

The rest of the cardiovascular system is made up of blood vessels. There are three basic types of blood vessels: *arteries*, which carry blood from the heart to the tissues; *capillaries*, which are the smallest vessels, where life-giving substances pass from the bloodstream to the tissues and from the tissues back to the bloodstream; and *veins*, which transport blood back to the heart.

Now we're going to *really* get advanced in our anatomy lesson. There are specialized arteries called *arterioles*, through which blood passes just before it gets to the capillaries. Arterioles are important because they constantly change size, acting as "gatekeepers" to control exactly where the blood flows, to where it is needed the most.

For example, after you eat, the arterioles to the stomach and intestines enlarge, allowing more blood to help in digestion. At the same time, the arterioles to your muscles clamp down. And at other times, when you exercise, the arterioles to the arms and legs dilate, or enlarge, delivering added oxygen to the muscles. So it's obvious that the arterioles are key to controlling blood pressure in the normal, day-to-day activities of your body. For that reason, the arterioles are key to the way many antihypertensive drugs work.

Is this why your mother used to tell you not to go swimming after you ate?

Your blood pressure is always changing. That's because what you are doing is different from minute to minute. Like when you exercise. In order to deliver more blood to the muscles, the heart pumps more forcefully. This drives the blood pressure higher than it was just seconds before, when you were inactive. And when you argue with

These changes in blood vessel size are due to the **autonomic nervous system.** This is a network of nerves, outside of our conscious control, found among the brain, spinal cord, organs, and blood vessels. The part of this group of nerves involved with blood pressure is called the **sympathetic nervous system.** Drugs that block these nerves in treating hypertension are called **sympatholytics.**

your brother-in-law, it goes even higher as your body leaps from tranquillity to hostility. But when you are asleep, except for digesting that unfortunate midnight feeding of Mama Carlone's grand supreme pizza, your tissues need far less fuel to function than they did during the day. So at night, the blood pressure falls. And that's how it goes throughout the day and night, the blood pressure constantly adjusting to your body's changing needs.

This brings us to two very important points, which you'll hear again. First, *a blood pressure reading has a lot more meaning when the time of day and activity are recorded at the same time.* Second, *temporary blood pressure elevations due to increased activity are normal, and do not imply that those activities need to be avoided* (although we might quibble about the midnight pizza).

As you can see, you are a lot more complicated than the municipal waterworks, which must maintain only one pressure to deliver water to the kitchen sink. In contrast, your body has to constantly change the blood pressure as it copes with all sorts of bodily positions, conditions, and activities. And these changes must take place in *seconds*.

How does your body do this?

It starts with an incredible network of sensors, called *baroreceptors*. These sensors continuously monitor the pressure inside the arteries, sending a steady stream of information to the brain. The brain constantly analyzes these signals coming from the blood vessels and other sources, just as your eyes would spot a bear coming from behind a bush.

The brain reacts to all this data by signaling the heart to either speed up and pump harder (raise the BP) or to slow down and pump with less force (lower the BP). At the same time, the brain sends nerve impulses to the adrenal gland, which releases blood

> **Baroreceptors** are special nerve endings located in the walls of certain large arteries near the heart. Second by second, the baroreceptors monitor the pressure inside the arteries and transmit this information, by way of the autonomic nervous system, to the brain and heart.

pressure–controlling hormones such as adrenaline into the circulation.

This intricate, fascinating system of signals from the blood vessels to the brain, and from the brain back to the heart, glands, and blood vessels, is known as the sympathetic nervous system, and it's the way your body maintains just the right pressure for your needs at all times.

Puts the waterworks to shame, doesn't it?

Two Blood Pressures?

Yes, your blood pressure is really *two* blood pressures, and *both* are important. We used to say that only the "lower" pressure mattered. However, we now know that this is not true. Every blood pressure reading consists of two numbers: the *systolic* (pronounced "sis-tall-ic") pressure and the *diastolic* (pronounced "dye-iss-tall-ic") pressure. Both pressures are measured each time the blood pressure is taken. You can't have one without the other.

The systolic pressure is the highest pressure, generated by the pumping action of each heartbeat. When the heart contracts, blood is pushed forward, out of the heart and into the arteries, causing a wave of pressure spreading through every artery in the body.

The diastolic pressure is the lowest pressure in the arteries. It occurs between each heartbeat, when the heart is relaxed and refilling with blood as it prepares for the next beat. However, because there is *always* some pressure inside the arteries, blood still flows forward during diastole—just with not as much vigor as during systole.

When the blood pressure is taken, the systolic pressure is measured first and recorded on top. The diastolic pressure is measured second and recorded on the bottom. A typical reading is written 120/80, and is read "one-twenty over eighty." So, the first number, "120," is the systolic blood pressure, the pressure inside the arteries when your heart contracts. The second number, "80," is the diastolic pressure, the pressure when the heart is relaxed.

120—**systolic**
80—**diastolic**

The standard arm blood pressure measures the pressure within the *brachial artery*, the large artery you can feel pulsating on the inside of your elbow. The other location where doctors sometimes measure the blood pressure is over arteries in the lower extremities, where the systolic pressure is 20mm to 30mm Hg higher than in the arms. (That "mm Hg" is the unit measure for BP. We'll explain what it means in chapter 2.) The diastolic pressure is about the same in both upper and lower extremities.

The blood pressure is a measure of the pressure in the arteries during a *single* heartbeat. If the doctor enters the room carrying a syringe attached to a two-foot needle, your eyes may send a distress signal to the brain. In turn, your brain informs your heart to start pumping hard enough to allow you to make a fast exit from the room if you choose to do so. Suddenly the blood pressure is considerably higher. This relates to something we call "white-coat hypertension" which we'll talk about later.

It is never enough to rely on any *one* blood pressure measurement to determine whether you have hypertension at all, how bad it is, or whether treatment is working.

Another note about "normal" blood pressure. As wonderful as the body is at regulating the blood pressure, the system can become overwhelmed. For example, everyone, at times, carries more blood than we should. Like after eating Mama Carlone's salt-saturated pizza, which can raise a lot of folks' blood pressure. And everybody is tense at times too, like when stepping on the scale after eating Mama Carlone's pizza; this raises the pressure even more. However, *such temporary rises alone are not real hypertension.* Although pizza-type BP elevations shouldn't be disregarded, they are no reason to panic either. Remember: blood pressure normally fluctuates according to the state of your body and mind.

Aside from what you're doing and thinking, the time of day itself affects blood pressure. It changes a lot as you pass through each twenty-four-hour period, even more so in older people. This is part of your body's *circadian rhythm*. The blood pressure is normally highest about 9:00 in the morning, staying at that level until mid-afternoon. At about 3:00 P.M. it starts to fall, reaching a low point around 1:00 A.M. It remains low for a few hours, until just before awakening. Around 5:00 A.M. it climbs sharply back up toward its 9:00 A.M. peak. Then the whole cycle repeats itself. This pattern is the same both for people with and without hypertension; the only difference is that people with uncontrolled hypertension have higher pressures at any particular time.

Circadian Rhythm: the body's natural 24-hour rhythm of biological activities

That's why, when we suspect that hypertension may be present, we insist on repeated measurements, under very well-defined conditions, possibly at different times of the day. This is the best way to judge whether hypertension is truly present, and how bad it really is.

Finally, a word about *low* blood pressure. Unless there is a serious problem, like a heart attack, a very slow heartbeat, or considerable blood loss, there's nothing wrong with it. In fact, low everyday blood pressure when there is no other condition present has been found to relate to a lower risk for cardiovascular complications later in life.

Now let's explore hypertension.

What Causes Hypertension?

First, let's consider *primary hypertension*. Its exact cause is unknown, but we believe at least part of the answer is hidden in the genes.

Why do we suspect this? Very often many members of the same family have hypertension. Medical scientists believe that this probably occurs via a genetic code that sets blood pressure higher than is healthy, like you can set a house thermostat for a temperature that's too hot for comfort. The result is that your body works to keep your blood pressure higher than you need. For any given activity or at any time of day, the blood pressure is too high.

There are plenty of other theories about the cause of primary hypertension. But until the scientists agree, we'll spare you the details. Fortunately, *we don't have to know the cause to successfully treat primary hypertension.*

We have a lot better understanding of *secondary hypertension.* This form of hypertension is due to another disease resulting in the release of various hormones into the bloodstream. These hormones overstimulate the heartbeat and constrict the arteries so much that the blood pressure goes up.

What causes secondary hypertension? Here is a partial list:

Acromegally

Adrenal gland disease

Brain tumors

Carcinoid disease

Coarctation of the aorta

Hypercalcemia

Kidney disease

Pheochromocytoma

Porphyria

Sleep apnea

Spinal cord lesions

Thyroid disease

In addition to diseases, many medications can also elevate the blood pressure. We will have more to say about those in chapter 5.

Another Reason to Stay Out of the Candy Store

A very rare cause of secondary hypertension is a glandular disorder in which eating licorice is the culprit. Licorice? Yep—here's the explanation, right from the doctors' own textbook: "The glyccyrrhizic acid in licorice inhibits the 11b-OH-dehydrogenase enzyme responsible for conversion of cortisol, which exerts potent mineralocoricoid action in the kidney, to cortisone, which is much less potent, thereby inducing 'apparent' mineralocorticoid excess." (From *Internal Medicine,* 3rd edition, Jay H. Stein, editor.)

Who Gets Hypertension?

People of either sex, at any age, and with any ethnic and socioeconomic background. Some people, however, are more likely than others to become hypertensive. These folks include:

- African-Americans, who are twice as likely to get hypertsion as Caucasians, and tend to have more serious degrees of hypertension.

- People with a family history of hypertension.
- People with certain other conditions, such as diabetes, gout, lipid disorders, and obesity.

What about Stress?

The sixty-four-zillion-dollar question that everybody always asks about hypertension is what this has to do with "stress." After all, it is called hyper*tension*, isn't it? Doesn't stress reside in the brain, which helps control blood pressure? And doesn't stress elevate the blood pressure?

True, true, and true. But temporary blood pressure elevation caused by stress is not the same as hypertension. It is just an uncomfortable part of our survival instinct.

Let's pretend you are out in the woods, taking photos of birds. It is very tranquil. Your heart beats calmly. Your muscles are relaxed, needing little oxygen. As you would expect, the blood pressure is low.

Suddenly, a bear lumbers out from behind a bush. Your once-placid cardiovascular system jolts into action (thanks to your sympathetic nervous system), shoving your blood pressure and heart-beat into the stratosphere.

Why does the body react like this? It's what we call preparing for "fight or flight." This is another way to say that, when you sense danger, your muscles are suddenly fed the oxygen they need to propel you to safety (or, if you'd rather, to battle the bear).

Although this sort of situation may have been common among ancient cave dwellers, most twentieth-century stress is not due to bear encounters. Rather, our daily dangers are more the telephone-ringing, horn-honking, boss-fearing, bill-paying varieties of stress. None of which are directly life-threatening, but the brain doesn't know how else to react to something it perceives as a bad situation. So it readies you for "fight or flight," and up goes the blood pressure.

This is an unhealthy response of the BP that some of us have worse than others. And, to a certain extent, we can learn to control it. But the main point is this: *Occasional blood pressure elevations like this don't mean you have hypertension.*

So, what about stress as a cause of hypertension?

- First, there is no good evidence that stress itself *causes* hypertension.

- Second, blood pressure elevation during stress is to be expected.

- Third, *no* blood pressure elevation should be ignored and attributed to mere "nerves," until repeat measurements during nonstressful times have been made.

- Finally, if you have hypertension, sustained or frequent stress can make blood pressure control more difficult to achieve.

What about Weight?

Excess weight causes some changes in body metabolism that also elevate blood pressure. As a result, obesity can make hypertension a lot worse. That's why weight loss is one of the most effective nondrug treatments for hypertension.

Salt?

Important question. Salt comes in many forms. The one we're most concerned about in hypertension is *sodium chloride.* That's what you find in good old salt water, which is mostly what blood is made up of (remember our little sea creature who wanted to live on land?). So if you ingest too much sodium, your blood pressure *might* go up—it depends on your metabolism. Like stress and obesity, sodium is especially likely to elevate your blood pressure if you have hypertension, borderline hypertension, or even high normal blood pressure.

There are other forms of salt, like potassium, calcium, and magnesium. The final word isn't in on these, although some people with abnormally *low* potassium levels tend to run a little higher blood pressure. There is also some weak evidence that low calcium and magnesium levels are somehow related to high blood pressure as well. But most experts don't believe that deficiencies of these salts cause hypertension.

So What's Happening?

Hopefully, we've convinced you by now that a normal blood pressure is whatever your body needs to function effectively and safely, whether it's digesting food or running from bears.

What, then, is going on when you have hypertension?

Researchers have found that there are at least three different ways that hypertension can come about. This information will also help us understand how various drugs work to control high blood pressure.

Too Much Water in the Bloodstream

First, there can be more circulating blood than the cardiovascular system was designed to handle. Consider what would happen if everyone in the city stopped using water, but the pumps at the municipal waterworks kept forcing water into the system. Inevitably the water pressure would rise.

Now, let's suppose that a hormone tells your kidneys to stop getting rid of as much water as you drink. Because blood is mostly water, the amount of blood (normally about four quarts) circulating in your cardiovascular system would increase, and along with it, your blood pressure.

This is one reason why diuretics work so well in hypertension. Diuretics rid the body of salt and water, mostly through the kidneys. This shrinks the blood volume, thereby lowering the blood pressure.

The Big Squeeze

The second way the blood pressure goes up in hypertension is via what doctors call *increased peripheral resistance*. This occurs when the small arteries, mainly the arterioles, narrow too much.

Consider, again, your water supply. Let's pretend that the city installs all new water mains, but they make a mistake: the new mains are smaller than the old ones. Now those big pumps at the

> **Peripheral Resistance:**
> The force that blood being pumped by the heart has to over-come in order to get to the tissues. (Don't worry about it—most medical students don't understand it, either.)

water station are forcing the same amount of water through a narrower system of pipes. What happens? The pressure in the city water system goes up, turning your showerhead into a cannon.

Same thing in your body. In hypertension, the arterioles squeeze down more than they should, while your heart continues pumping the same amount of blood but through arteries that now have a smaller capacity. As a result, the BP goes up.

This explains how other types of BP medications work. By relaxing the arterioles, the cardiovascular system's capacity enlarges, and the BP comes back down.

Pumping with Power

The third way the blood pressure can go up in hypertension is for the heart to pump blood with more force than it should. Doctors have labeled this *increased cardiac output,* occurring due to *increased sympathetic activity.*

Remember what the brain does when you see a bear in the woods? Via the sympathetic nervous system it tells the heart to pump harder and faster. The sudden increase in the heart's power as it pumps blood causes a surge in the blood pressure.

> **Cardiac Output:**
> The amount of blood being pumped by the heart.

For this reason, drugs that block the activity of the sympathetic nervous system are particularly effective.

All of the Above

Although these are three different ways that blood pressure goes up in hypertension, they are often *all* present, in varying degrees, in some people. If one way predominates, then those types of drugs that act to reverse that particular effect tend to work best. This also explains why it's sometimes desirable to use more than one type of drug to lower blood pressure.

What's So Bad about Hypertension?

The football teams under a famous coach were known for seldom throwing a forward pass. One day a sportswriter asked the coach why he didn't like to pass. He replied that he didn't like the odds, because when you threw the football three things could happen, and two of them were bad. The same is true for the odds of uncontrolled hypertension, with one basic difference: the stakes are higher than the outcome of a football game.

For Those of You Who Know Nothing about Football:
1. The pass can be completed, which is GOOD.
2. The pass can be dropped, which is BAD.
3. The pass can be intercepted, which is VERY BAD.

What happens when your hypertension goes untreated?

First, maybe nothing. You could live to a ripe old age. Problem is, your insurance carrier won't bet on that. You shouldn't either.

Second, the hypertension may keep getting worse, making later treatment much more difficult.

Third, several very serious, life-threatening complications are much more likely to occur. These are worth taking a closer look at:

Stroke: The medical term is *cerebrovascular accident (CVA)*, and it can occur two ways: through blockage of a blood vessel to the brain by fatty deposits called atherosclerosis; or bleeding into the brain, called a *subarachnoid hemorrhage* when the bleeding is on the surface of the brain and *intracerebral hemorrhage* when the bleeding is directly into the brain itself.

Cerebro = brain
Vascular = blood vessel

Heart attack: Called *myocardial infarction (MI)* by doctors, this is also caused by atherosclerosis of the coronary arteries, which supply blood to the heart.

Myocardial = heart muscle
Infarction = sudden loss of blood supply
During a myocardial infarct, a portion of the myocardium—the heart muscle itself—dies due to a blockage of an artery supplying the muscle with oxygen and nutrients. The amount of muscle that is lost may be large or small. Myocardial infarction is the leading killer of both men and women in the United States.

Heart failure: The heart muscle thickens, the heart chambers enlarge, and the heart literally "wears out" due to years of pumping against high pressure.

Kidney failure: The kidneys, especially small areas called *glomeruli* whose job is to filter the blood as it forms urine, "wear out" from years of pounding from the high pressures.

> **Glomeruli:**
> In Latin, glomus translates to "ball," which is what the glomeruli resemble: balls or clusters of blood vessels that project into the ends of the tubes that transport urine from the kidney.

Arterial aneurysm: "Ballooning" of the walls of the large arteries, especially the aorta, due to weakening from high pressures combined with atherosclerosis.

> **Aneurysm:**
> In Greek, aneurysma translates to "a widening." The walls of the artery, weakened by disease, such as hypertension, actually expand, forming a sac that fills with blood.

Peripheral vascular disease: Blockage of arteries to the legs by atherosclerosis.

Not exactly a dropped forward pass, is it?

Is There Any Good News?

Yes! Controlling hypertension is *extremely* effective in preventing all of these complications.

Can Hypertension Be Prevented?

We're not sure. But, in some people, lifestyle changes can delay the onset of hypertension, perhaps for many years.

How do we do this? By paying close attention to the different factors that help lead to hypertension in the first place.

First, let's look at the factors that you can't change, but which you should be aware of, alerting you to the increased possibility of hypertension. The uncontrollable risk factors are:

Heredity

Hypertension runs in families. If your grandmother, grandfather, mother, father, brother, sister, son, or daughter has it, the chances are increased that you'll get it, too. And the more of them who have it, the greater likelihood you will have hypertension. (But you also could be the only person in your family, right through the most distant cousin, to have hypertension.)

Age

This is a little confusing. There's no question that hypertension is more common as people get older. Over 60 percent of folks over age sixty-five have hypertension.

So what's the mystery about relating age and hypertension? Just this: An increasing blood pressure is not an *automatic* part of the aging process. After all, people also gain weight and stop exercising as they get older. These factors, unlike birthdays, are usually controllable. Some things we don't like about getting older are our own fault.

Ethnic Groups

No race is spared from hypertension. In the United States, African-Americans are more commonly afflicted than others. Whether this is purely due to genetics, or to lifestyle differences, such as diet, isn't certain. The disease also begins at a younger age and tends to be more severe in African-Americans, especially men. For these reasons, African-Americans with untreated hypertension are also more likely to suffer from strokes, heart attacks, and kidney disease.

Next, let's take a brief look at some of the factors contributing to hypertension that we definitely *can* do something about. The controllable risk factors are:

Weight

People with lower weights have lower pressures.

Alcohol

May be a "sedative" to your brain, but *not* to your cardiovascular system, where it directly elevates the blood pressure; also contains lots of calories and is a terrific appetite stimulant—in other words, helps put the weight on, too.

Exercise

Sedentary folks have higher blood pressures than active folks.

Dietary sodium

Overall, salt lovers have higher BPs too.

One more thing. To be perfectly honest, you can lead a "perfect" life and become hypertensive. But doing the right things, like keeping your weight down, exercising, and reducing your sodium intake might help delay its onset. And when it does occur, these lifestyle habits will probably make the treatment a lot easier, even lessening the chances of complications like stroke and heart attack from happening later.

Does It Ever Go Away?

Once hypertension is *truly* present, no.

Occasionally, people who have been on blood pressure medications for a long time can maintain a normal blood pressure for a while off all drugs. But it almost always goes back up after several months, or even a few years.

The blood pressure can also fall to normal with weight reduction. But the disease of hypertension will always remain, ready to push the pressure back up if weight is regained. So there's really only one way we should look at hypertension: It is a lifelong disease that needs control for a lifetime.

It's Your Turn

1. Do you have any immediate family members with hypertension?
   - ❑ Mother or father*
   - ❑ Brother or sister*
   - ❑ Children*

2. Are you over age 65?
   - ❑ Yes   ❑ No

3. Are you overweight?
   - ❑ Yes*   ❑ No

4. Do you drink alcohol?
   - ❑ Yes*   ❑ No

5. Are you physically inactive?
   - ❑ Yes*   ❑ No

6. Do you usually add salt to your food after it is cooked?
   - ❑ Yes*   ❑ No

*Discuss this with your doctor if you haven't already done so.

2

Do You Have Hypertension?

MANY OF THE sixty million people in the United States who have hypertension don't even know it. And some people who believe they have hypertension, even take medications for it, don't really have hypertension. *Both are very dangerous situations that must be avoided.*

In the Beginning . . .

Once upon a time, in a shopping mall . . . or at a health fair . . . or in a health clinic for a preemployment examination . . . you were first told your blood pressure was elevated.

Thanks to a massive, nationwide effort spearheaded by organizations such as the American Heart Association several years ago, everybody . . . well, almost everybody . . . can't help but have their blood pressure taken now and then. It seems like almost anywhere you go somebody is ready to pump up a cuff around your arm.

Even dentist offices got into the act. Dentists? Is it so surprising that your blood pressure might be elevated as you watch your dentist, the most feared creature to roam the earth since *Tyrannosaurus rex*, prepare to explore the inside of your mouth with a stainless steel pick?

Just what, you ask, is your blood pressure *supposed* to be in shopping malls, fairs, and Dr. Rex's chamber of oral horrors? After all, you're only human, right?

Right. We don't really know exactly what dental and other BPs

mm Hg?

Once upon a time, in some remote civilization, lived a strange scientist. As an expert in measuring the pressures of things, he figured out one day how he could confuse people forever, so that only he would ever really understand what "pressure" was. It was simple: pressures would be measured by how high they pushed mercury up a thin glass column. To add to the confusion, the scientist plotted, the height of the mercury would be measured in millimeters. To this day, BP is stated in millimeters (abbreviated "mm") of mercury (abbreviated "Hg"), written as "mm Hg."

should be—certainly at least a little higher than when you're reading a book on gardening beside a lazy stream. But what we do know is that if it's over 140mm Hg systolic or over 90mm Hg diastolic, you *could* have hypertension, or at least be on the road to hypertension sometime in the future. Elevated pressures, regardless of the circumstances, *must be taken seriously* and followed up. Tens of thousands of people owe their good health to blood pressure screening by the Dr. Rex's of the world.

Who Do You See?

Easy. If you're told your blood pressure is high, make an appointment with your personal physician (family practitioner, internist, pediatrician, etc.), who is trained and experienced in the diagnosis and treatment of hypertension.

What about a "hypertension specialist"? While some physicians may limit their practices to treating hypertension, no such formal specialty exists. The closest would be a *nephrologist*, a kidney specialist, because the kidney is so intimately involved in regulating the blood pressure, and many kidney diseases cause hypertension.

When your personal physician suspects a rare cause of hypertension, or when treatment doesn't respond the way it should, you may be referred to another physician, such as a nephrologist. You may also be referred to another physician specializing in treating specific organs that can be damaged by hypertension, such as a cardiologist if your heart is involved.

Nephro = Kidney
Nephrologist: a physician who specializes in treating kidney disorders.

The Initial Evaluation

Once hypertension is suspected, there are three initial tasks:

- First, to determine whether you really have hypertension. (This may take time.)
- Second, to look for target organ damage.
- Third, to establish whether you have other risk factors for cardiovascular disease.

This evaluation should not be put off, with one exception: if you are in the midst of some truly exceptional, temporary crisis or turmoil in your life, which can affect the blood pressure. Under these circumstances, your physician may decide to defer an evaluation for a while. So it's important to tell your physician about any unusual problems going on in your life. But once this has passed, you should seek a definitive answer about whether you have hypertension.

Never automatically assume *any* blood pressure elevation is stress-related.

Making the Diagnosis

The diagnosis of hypertension is usually based upon readings obtained in the doctor's office.

Here are some general rules the doctor follows to get the most accurate and meaningful BPs (watch how they do it, because you may be taking your own BP at home, as we discuss in chapter 5):

- You should not have smoked or drunk caffeine within thirty minutes.

- You should be seated with your arm bared and supported at about the level of your heart (unless you've had a heart transplant to your leg or some other unusual location, this is about the center of the chest).

- Measurements begin about five minutes after being seated.

- Appropriate cuff size should be used—if too small, the reading may be falsely high; if too large, the reading may be falsely low.

- Both the systolic and diastolic pressures should be recorded.

- Two or more readings should be taken. These should be separated by at least two minutes, then averaged. If the first two readings differ by more than 5 mm Hg, additional readings should be obtained.

In addition, you may notice that the doctor takes the BP in both arms, maybe even in the thigh. That's to check for a cause of secondary hypertension called *coarctation of the aorta*.

Now let's look at some general guidelines for interpreting the *initial* readings:

Coarctation of the Aorta:
A birth defect involving the aorta, the major artery leaving the heart. The narrowing causes the blood pressure to be higher in the right arm than in the left arm, or higher in the arms than in the legs, depending on the location of the defect.

- If the BP is over 160/100, you almost certainly have hypertension. The doctor may want more measurements, perhaps taken outside the office, before making any final decisions about treatment. You will also receive a full medical evaluation. If the BP is very high, you may be started on medications immediately.
- If the BP is 120/80 or under, you don't have hypertension.
- If the BP is any combination of pressures in the range of 125–160/85–100, your doctor will probably make additional measurements over the next few weeks before deciding the next course of action.

Most folks with suspected hypertension fall into this third category. But you're wondering: If the BP is up, even a little, why doubt the readings taken in the doctor's office? *Because as many as one in five persons would be falsely diagnosed as having hypertension if only office BPs were used.*

This is because of something called "white-coat hypertension."

"White-Coat Hypertension"

Doctors usually wear white coats, although blues and grays and even occasional pinks and yellows can be seen darting in and out of clinic treatment rooms. But regardless of the color, some people's psyches truly panic when confronted by a doctor. Like running into a bear in the woods, these folks suddenly experience "flight or fight," and up goes their BP.

When this happens to you, there is a dilemma. How can you ever find out whether you truly have hypertension when your doctor reminds you of Ol' Grizzly?

White-Coat Wars

While it may seem like a pretty boring topic to most of us, one of the most heated disagreements among hypertension experts today is the value of ambulatory monitoring. Opinions vary from its being a meaningless waste of money to the only way to be sure whether a person actually has hypertension.

First, they will try to get you to relax, right there in the office, despite all those horrible things your doctor has done to you in the past. For example, they might try turning off the lights and playing soft music.

If all efforts at tranquillity fail to bring the BP down, the next step will probably be to have you return one or more times, to have it checked again by the doctor or nurse.

Another option is to have your pressure recorded by *ABPM* (ambulatory blood pressure monitoring). ABPM consists of having a portable device attached to your arm and connected to a miniature tape recorder. This gives a continuous measure of your BP for twenty-four hours. The idea is to find out what your blood pressure is under a variety of circumstances, including periods of supposed calm, as opposed to the ghastly environs of a doctor's office. The main problem with ABPM is cost. Your doctor may have to convince your health plan that it's really necessary.

The best solution may be for you to take your own BP. There's a good chance that you'll be doing this anyway, assuming you do have high blood pressure. Which means, of course, that you'll have to buy a BP measuring device and learn how to use it. We have a lot to say about that in chapter 5.

Back to the Numbers

Now we've collected all these BPs, and you and your doctor are satisfied that they represent the real you. Here's what they mean:

 Optimal blood pressure is a systolic pressure of less than 120mm Hg and a diastolic of less than 80mm Hg. This is the range that puts you in the lowest possible risk for complications, compared with other people of your age, gender, and ethnic background.

Normal blood pressure is considered to be a systolic pressure of less than 130mm Hg, and a diastolic of less than 85mm Hg. This is the range in which the BP doesn't carry a risk for complications any greater than for the average population. Which means, of course, that it's still possible to have a stroke or one of the many other problems commonly associated with hypertension, but researchers tell us that lowering your blood pressure from this level doesn't further reduce your risks.

High normal blood pressure refers to a systolic pressure from 130mm Hg to 139mm Hg and a diastolic pressure from 85mm Hg to 89mm Hg. Pressures in this range carry a slightly increased risk for complications, but the risk is not great enough to justify drug therapy. However, these BPs should be monitored closely in the future. Definite hypertension sometimes occurs later, particularly if you do something really stupid like gain (maybe even a little) weight. Risk modification, such as lowering your cholesterol, exercising regularly, quitting smoking, losing weight, and cutting back on alcohol, are all strongly advised. We'll cover these in detail in chapter 3.

Hypertension means the systolic pressure is 140mm Hg or greater, or the diastolic pressure is 90mm Hg or greater. Such pressures are clearly abnormal and are associated with increased risk of complications.

A special note here, on *systolic hypertension.* It used to be thought that the elevation of systolic pressure (140mm Hg and over) with a normal diastolic pressure (under 90mm Hg) was okay. But we know better now. An elevation of the systolic pressure alone is hypertension, too, and *should be treated when the systolic pressure is 160 or greater.* This is a common problem in older folks.

Staging

We used to label hypertension as "mild," "moderate," and "severe." The problem with that way of thinking was that folks told they had "mild" hypertension sometimes breathed a big sigh of relief, didn't take their medications, and later on had a stroke or some other complication that was anything but "mild." Regardless of the numbers, *all hypertension should be taken seriously.*

As a result, *JNC V* came up with a new way of classifying hypertension, so no one would be misled. The new classification placed hypertension into *stages.*

	Systolic BP (mm Hg)	Diastolic BP (mm Hg)
Stage 1	140–159	90–99
Stage 2	160–179	100–109
Stage 3	180–209	110–119
Stage 4	210 or greater	120 or greater

What do these stages mean? With each increase in stage, the blood pressure is more likely to cause target organ damage and complications. BPs in higher stages are also more difficult to bring down to normal levels, requiring stronger medications. And Stages 3 and 4 can even cause symptoms, although even these levels tend to remain "silent."

The Next Step

If your BPs fall into *any* stage of hypertension, and maybe if you fall into the high normal category as well, your doctor's next step will be to perform an evaluation (history, physical, laboratory tests) to determine:

- Whether target organ damage is present. This is mainly concerned with the blood vessels, the kidneys, and the heart.

- Whether you have any other risk factors for cardio-vascular disease.

- Whether you have the primary or secondary form of hypertension.

The History

Some of the questions you'll need to answer are aimed at:

- Episodes of severe BP elevations, such as headache, tiredness, light-headedness, sweating, palpitations, chest discomfort (if present, these point to the possibility of secondary hypertension).

- Your personal history, family history, and symptoms of kidney disease, heart disease, stroke, diabetes mellitus, and lipid (cholesterol) abnormalities.

- Past trauma, especially to the flanks (could cause kidney damage).

- Recent weight gain or loss.
- Use of tobacco and alcohol.
- Cocaine or other substance abuse.

Coke (as in Cocaine)
In addition to frying the brain and raising blood pressure, cocaine use, by any route, causes an encyclopedia of health problems. Here are a few: heart attack, irregular heartbeat, enlargement of the heart, rupture of the stomach and intestines, blindness, seizures, strokes, rupture and bleeding of the lungs, spontaneous abortion, massive destruction of the muscles, impotence, and sudden death.

- Eating habits, including special diets, salt intake (e.g., you eat an entire Mama Carlone's pizza at least once a week), and fat consumption.
- Exercise habits, with any noticeable change in strength or endurance.
- Sleeping habits, with any recent change (snoring can be important—see chapter 3).
- Emotional status (e.g., feelings of depression or unusual anxiety, for any reason).
- Medications, taken regularly or intermittently, including both prescription and nonprescription (over the counter).

The Physical

The physical examination is "complete," depending on when you last had any sort of evaluation. Hypertension doesn't involve just the arm—it affects every part of the body. Here's what the doctor will pay special attention to:

- **Skin:** color, thickness, temperature, hair loss.
- **Eyes:** for signs of hypertension, such as narrowed arteries and even small hemorrhages caused by elevated pressure, by looking directly at the back of the eyes (the retina) through a handheld instrument called an ophthalmoscope.

- **Large arteries:** for signs of blockage of arteries to the brain (the *carotid* arteries, in the neck); to the kidneys (the *renal* arteries, the flanks); to the abdominal organs (the *aorta*—also whether it is dilated); and to the lower extremities (the *iliac* and *femoral* arteries, the groin and thigh).

- **Heart:** for evidence of enlargement or changes in its pumping action.

- **Abdomen:** for tumor masses and enlargement of organs.

- **Legs:** for edema and skin ulcers.

Skin Color?

Several gland disorders can cause secondary hypertension, such as thyroid and adrenal disease. These also make the skin tan, due to an overabundance of a hormone called melanin.

Tests

These days everybody is keeping a close eye on costs, especially when it comes to performing tests. Unless there's a good reason for a test, your doctor isn't going to order it.

Certain tests are considered important to everyone with hypertension. They are useful in screening for secondary forms of hypertension such as kidney disease; for commonly associated diseases, such as diabetes; for target organ damage that may have already occurred, such as heart disease; for other risk factors, such as lipid abnormalities; and for giving your doctor key baseline measurements that will become important in planning and monitoring drug therapy, such as the potassium and uric acid.

These "routine" tests are:

- Blood glucose (ideally done after not eating for several hours)
- Calcium
- Complete blood count (CBC)
- Creatinine
- Electrocardiogram
- Lipids (total cholesterol, HDL, triglycerides)
- Potassium
- Uric acid
- Urinalysis

Test$

Anyone who has ever had the courage to figure out a medical bill (and worse yet, pay it), knows that many tests must be intended for Arab sheiks and NFL quarterbacks. Despite the desirability of owning one's personal counterfeiting machine to pay for them, certain tests, if used with wisdom and discretion, are very valuable and often essential. Just be sure to talk to your doctor about exactly how they are going to help your evaluation. The final decision in any testing is always yours.

Your doctor may want to perform additional tests, based on the initial evaluation. For example, if your heart appears to be enlarged, you may have a chest X ray and an echocardiogram to determine the size of the heart. Or if kidney abnormalities are suspected, imaging tests (like X rays) of the kidneys and more detailed analysis of the urine may be carried out.

Planning Treatment

By now, your doctor has a lot of information about you, your blood pressure, and the organs most likely to be harmed by hypertension.

As you can see, there are so many factors that come into play that there really is no "medical cookbook" your doctor can open up to learn exactly what's going to work best for you.

This is a good example of why doctors call this the "practice of medicine." Every patient is different, and every treatment is a little different as well. Just like buying a suit, a general size gets you and the tailor started, but the perfect fit is made only with precise measurements that are unique to you and to no one else in the world.

Before We Move On

After two chapters, hypertension may appear to be a pretty dismal disease. Left untreated, it can be.

But the truth is also that the rest of this book is good news, because treatment really works, given a little understanding and desire to take control on your part.

That's why your active involvement is a key element to success.

It's Your Turn

1. Is your personal doctor a:

❑ Family practitioner

❑ Internist

❑ Pediatrician

❑ Obstetrician-gynecologist

❑ Other:_____

2. If you are on blood pressure medications, what was your average BP before starting treatment?

Systolic: _____*   Diastolic: _____*

3. What stage of hypertension do you have?*

❑ 1   ❑ 2   ❑ 3   ❑ 4

4. What type of hypertension do you have?*

❑ Primary   ❑ Secondary

Cause:_____

5. Do you have abnormalites on any of the following blood tests?*

❑ Blood cell count

❑ Calcium

❑ Cathecholamines

❑ Cholesterol or other blood fats—list:

_____

❑ Creatinine

❑ Glucose

❑ Potassium

❑ Uric acid

❑ Other

6. Do you have abnormalities of any of the following other tests?*

    ❑ Urinalysis

    ❑ Chest X ray

    ❑ Echocardiogram

    ❑ Other—list:

_____

*Ask your doctor if you don't know the answer.

3

What Can You Do for Yourself?

THE KEY TO TAKING control over any chronic condition like hypertension is first accepting it as part of your life, then dealing with it accordingly. Like driving in rush-hour traffic, listening to your boss's complaints, and paying bills, hypertension is an unwanted part of your life that you have to live with. The big difference is that unlike clogged freeways, grumpy bosses, and your spouse's credit card habits, *you really can do something about hypertension.*

It starts with learning everything you can about hypertension. Like taking this journey through *Ask the Doctor.* Then referring back to this "BP travel guide" when new questions arise. And asking your doctor things you don't understand, which at first may be a lot. Don't be shy, because what you don't know *can* hurt you.

Now we're going to tell you how lifestyle changes can help lower your blood pressure and reduce other risk factors for cardiovascular disease. And make no mistake: lifestyle is important to cardiovascular health, especially if you have hypertension. This remains just as true even if you take antihypertensive medications.

Just how important is lifestyle? Consider this: if you have hypertension, your chances for getting coronary heart disease *double* if you also have abnormal blood fats. And they almost *quadruple* if you have abnormal blood fats, diabetes, and smoke cigarettes.

It's time to do something about that weight, and a lot of other things.

Diet

Weight

Everybody's favorite subject.

The bad news: extra pounds and elevated blood pressure go hand in hand. Being overweight markedly increases your chances for getting hypertension.

The good news: studies have shown that people who are overweight and lose 5 to 10 percent of their weight have a significant fall in blood pressure.

Some people with Stage 1 hypertension can actually avoid the need to go on BP medications by losing weight. Others, who are already on medications, are able to reduce their medication dosage with weight loss. And there have even been times when people who were more than just a few pounds overweight actually stopped medications altogether by shedding enough pounds!

Caution: Never reduce doses or stop medications without the approval and guidance of your doctor.

In addition to lowering the blood pressure, weight loss also improves the blood fats. Clothes fit better, too. And you'll sure feel better at your proper weight.

Bet you can hardly wait to start shedding those pounds.

Yes Virginia, There Is a Calorie

Regardless of the method, all weight loss and weight maintenance involves—you guessed it—the dreaded "c" word: calorie. We tend to think of a calorie as a quivering little mass hiding in our food just waiting to strike. Then we eat the little demon, and he races though our stomach and into the bloodstream, where he charges for the nearest chin, waist, or rear end. Once in his new home he explodes himself into a massive white glob to forever peer over, around, and through the shirt and pants that once fit.

It's not that way at all, of course. The calorie isn't a substance of any kind, rather a bundle of energy contained within foods. Scientists define one calorie as the quantity of heat required to raise the temperature of one kilogram of water by one degree Celsius. Doesn't seem quite as fearsome when you look at it like that, does it? Nevertheless, too many of them is one of your worst enemies, because they do count!

What this means for us is that every calorie eaten must be used by our bodies as energy, or it will be converted into fat. If we don't exercise, this means we only need about 1,800 calories a day. For every 2,800 calories we take in but fail to burn off, we gain approximately one pound. But—happily—for every 2,800 calories we burn off, we lose one pound.

Alcohol

So you thought that vodka was the greatest tranquilizer ever invented, perfect for soothing the old blood pressure? Hardly. Alcohol in beer, whiskey, wine, or any other form is a potent *stimulant* to the cardiovascular system. Which means that it *raises* the blood pressure. And you don't have to drink yourself into a semi-coma to do it, either.

But all is not lost. When alcohol intake is reduced, the blood pressure falls.

Recommendation for your BP: limit your intake to one ounce of ethanol per day—that's two ounces (1¹/₃ jigger) of hundred-proof whiskey, eight ounces (one glass) of wine, or twenty-four ounces (two cans) of beer.

What's a Proof?

"Spirit proof" is a U.S. standard of alcohol, which translates as follows: 100 proof equals 50 percent of ethanol alcohol by volume, of an alcoholic mixture at 60 degrees Fahrenheit. Sorry you asked?

Alcohol Does That?

You've also probably read that alcohol may afford some protection against coronary heart disease. Exactly how much alcohol is needed for this effect, and why this occurs, still has to be sorted out. (Possible reason: alcohol increases the HDL cholesterol, also known as the "good" cholesterol.) Comment: alcohol still kills far more people than it might help, even if this is true. If you don't drink, don't start.

Sodium

Most of us consume far more salt than we need.

Know how much sodium chloride (table salt) you really need? Only one-fourth of a teaspoon a day!

The main reason salt is added to our food is for food preservation. Like on ancient sailing ships before refrigeration. But somewhere along the way, Mama Carlone and the other people who manufacture and prepare our food let it get out of hand, helping to create a society of salt lovers. In fact, up to 80 percent of our daily salt consumption comes from processed foods.

Medical studies in which people have been given diets low in sodium showed that sometimes this *alone* can bring down the blood pressure. However, human beings' metabolisms vary greatly from person to person, so sodium doesn't affect everyone's blood pressure to the same degree. African-Americans and the elderly seem to be more sensitive to salt than others.

They Make the Dough with Seawater or What?
Average amount of sodium in pizza from four leading
pizza chains (2 slices):

	Sodium
Cheese	910 mg
Pepperoni	1,124 mg
Veggie	1,155 mg
Deep pan cheese	962 mg
Deep pan pepperoni	1,174 mg
Deep pan veggie	1,138 mg

And who ever eats just two slices?

Do you use too much salt? Here's a quick quiz to help you decide:

- Do you salt your food at the table before tasting it? *If yes, you definitely eat too much salt.*

- Do you generally salt some of your food at the table after tasting it? *If yes, there's a good chance you eat too much salt.*

- Do you, or the person preparing the food, salt food only while cooking, according to taste? *If yes, you are probably not eating too much salt.*

Lesson: Ban saltshakers from the table.

The ABCs of Getting Salt Out of Your Food
Avoid chips, salted peanuts, pretzels, pickles, and ham.
Beware of processed and frozen foods.
Cut back on salt in your cooking.
Drive on by fast-food places.
Eat lots of fruits and vegetables.
Fix food with spices—meals might taste even better!
Get rid of the saltshaker from the table.
Have food labels on your mind when you shop.

If you complain that food just doesn't taste good unless it's encased in salt crystals, remember that you had to *learn* to like salt on your food, which means that this is one habit that can be *unlearned*. There are also plenty of creative ways to enhance food taste with herbs, spices, and various other ingredients that don't affect your blood pressure.

It's important to talk with your doctor about whether you should restrict your sodium intake to help control your blood pressure, and by how much.

Potassium

Ever see a chimpanzee with hypertension? Of course not! That's because they eat lots of bananas. We're kidding, of course—we don't really know much about BPs in chimps.

We do know, however, that bananas contain lots of potassium. People (and maybe monkeys) who eat a lot of foods high in potassium tend to run slightly lower blood pressures.

Fresh fruits and vegetables are loaded with potassium. Maybe even more important is that they're also low in fat, low in calories, and high in fiber. Which makes fruits and vegetables ideal foods in a lot of ways.

You can also get potassium in tablet form, but this is not recommended unless specifically ordered by your doctor, based on your blood potassium level. Reason: Potassium supplements have not proven beneficial in helping the blood pressure and they can cause the potassium to go too high, which is very dangerous. This can occur whenever we are unable to get rid of excess potassium from the body, which is the result of some kidney disorders or of taking potassium-sparing diuretics.

So play like a chimp and stick with bananas unless you're told otherwise.

Calcium

We're on less certain ground here, and wouldn't bring this up if there hadn't been so much written about calcium and hypertension.

Here's what we know. Calcium deficiency is associated with an increased incidence of hypertension, and a low calcium intake may worsen the effects of sodium on the blood pressure. Furthermore, increasing the amount of calcium in the diet of people with hypertension helps lower the pressure in some cases, but only a little bit.

Right now, our advice is that you get at least the minimum daily requirement of calcium (800 mg per day for men and non-lactating women), as far as your blood pressure is concerned. And regardless of your blood pressure, you should maintain a good calcium intake to help prevent osteoporosis, especially if you are a woman.

Magnesium

A lot has been written about magnesium, too. Bottom line: There's no convincing evidence you need to supplement your normal diet with magnesium for hypertension.

Fats

Fatty food doesn't directly affect your blood pressure. However, this is a critical part of your diet for you to control. This is why your doctor measured your cholesterol and other blood lipids when you were first found to have hypertension.

The reason is *atherosclerosis*. Although hypertension is bad in many ways, the number one problem is that it is a major factor in this buildup of the fatty deposits, fibrous tissue, and calcium in the walls of arteries. Atherosclerosis is the cause of almost all heart attacks and many strokes. So you can see how the combination of a fat-rich diet and hypertension is a prescription for real trouble.

And if that's not bad enough, dietary fats are also associated with colon cancer.

Vegetarian Diet

If you're a carnivore (that's a meat-eater), there's a good chance you've been made to feel guilty every time you bite into a chuck steak or a ham sandwich.

A vegetarian diet seems to help lower both the systolic and diastolic blood pressures. It also contains less fat and more dietary fiber (fiber itself has not been shown to lower the blood pressure, but has other benefits, such as lowering the risk of colon cancer), and more vegetable protein, calcium, and magnesium.

So why don't we all become vegetarians? That's fine for those who want to, provided nutritional deficiencies aren't created in the process. For the rest of us, we can still eat quite healthily with an occasional steak. Be sure to trim off the fat when you do.

Garlic and Onion

· Bad breath does not lower the blood pressure.

Fish Oil

Neither does bad taste and belching.

Caffeine

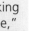

Two cups of coffee can raise the blood pressure as much as 15mm Hg. This effect can last for up to two hours. Despite this temporary rise in blood pressure, there is no evidence that caffeine itself either causes or worsens hypertension.

So enjoy your morning brew. In moderation, of course. And don't take your BP right away either—it could mislead you.

Enough for eating and drinking. Let's look at some other lifestyle issues.

> **Boiled Coffee?**
> In a study of people drinking "Scandinavian-style coffee," which is boiled, six cups per day increased the blood pressure. Shall we fry you a cup instead?

Tobacco

Just like caffeine, nicotine raises the blood pressure, normally for fifteen minutes or so. And we're not talking only about cigarettes here. *All* nicotine-containing tobacco raises the blood pressure. After the puff, drag, chew, or inhalation, the BP drops (unless another one is "enjoyed" in the meantime) back to where it was. Therefore, we can't truthfully say that smoking causes hypertension, or that quitting smoking will necessarily bring your blood pressure down to normal.

What we can say is that the main, truly devastating effect of tobacco on the cardiovascular system is that it is at least as destructive to your blood vessels, by promoting atherosclerosis, as hypertension. And the combination of the two together is another powerful prescription for future problems (yes, heart attack, stroke, kidney disease, etc.).

Nicotine also works against the effect of antihypertensive med-

Chew on This
Many cigarette smokers have decided that chewing tobacco is a safe substitute for kicking the habit. Wrong! Nicotine and the many other ingredients in chewing tobacco are absorbed from the mouth directly into the bloodstream, driving the BP straight through the stratosphere. It also causes mouth cancer. Of course, it does leave the teeth and gums looking nice, not to mention enhancing the breath.

ications. However, this may not be apparent by your usual blood pressure readings, if they are made when you haven't smoked for a while. For example, if you smoke, your blood pressure's probably higher away from the doctor's office—the reverse of "white-coat hypertension."

Finally, there is evidence that people with hypertension who smoke are much more likely to have their kidneys involved *(renovascular hypertension)* and to develop a very serious, rapidly progressive form of high blood pressure called *malignant hypertension.*

***Reno* = Kidney   *Vascular* = blood vessel**
Renovascular hypertension occurs when an artery to one of the kidneys becomes blocked, causing the kidney to release a hormone, called renin, that acts on other substances in the bloodstream to raise the blood pressure.

Just *quit.*

Exercise

Exercise is weird but wonderful. It seems to help almost everything a little bit, including lowering the blood pressure. On the average, being in good aerobic condition seems to lower the BP about 6–7mm Hg for both the systolic and diastolic pressures, even for people who aren't hypertensive. Folks with borderline hypertension may benefit the most.

Among people who exercise regularly, hypertension is less common (though it does occur). And the reverse is true. The more sedentary people are, the more likely they are to have hypertension.

In addition to allowing the body to function at a lower blood pressure, exercise has other indirect benefits in the control of hypertension. Weight is lower, anxiety is less, sleep is better, smoking cessation is easier. It also increases HDL cholesterol (the good cholesterol) and reduces what we call the blood viscosity (tendency of the blood to become sludgy)—kind of like the winterizing effect of special motor oils.

And of course, you just feel better when you are in good physical condition.

What kind of exercise? Anything that is sustained, ideally aerobic, from walking to gardening to bike riding. And, if you are inclined toward more vigorous activity like jogging, *and your doctor says okay* (you may need an exercise test first), go for it.

Calories Burned during Various Exercises	
Activity	*Cal/min*
Running (8mi/hr)	11
Cycling (13mi/hr)	10
Jogging (5mi/hr)	8
Tennis	7
Walking	7
Skating	6
Golf	
Carring clubs	5
Pulling cart	4
Riding cart	2
Bowling	4

Some people actually carry their golf clubs?

Unsustained, highly isometric exercises like weight lifting aren't beneficial. The blood pressure can actually rise to dangerous levels as you press three hundred pounds of dumbbells to the sky. So if you insist on bodybuilding, first obtain medical clearance.

We should also mention that some antihypertensive medications may make exercise a little more difficult. For example, beta-blockers can retard some folks' tolerance for exercise by their depressing effect on the heartbeat. By causing excess potassium loss, diuretics can hamper muscle function. And some of the more potent medications, like the adrenergic blockers, can cause the pressure to fall excessively after exercise.

One more thing. Don't undertake anything strenuous, beyond light activities such as walking, until your blood pressure is under control.

Medications

Many medications, both prescription and nonprescription, can elevate the blood pressure. They should either be stopped or, under your doctor's guidance, taken with extreme caution if there are no satisfactory alternatives.

You should always read the caution label on the box or the patient information sheet that comes with the prescription for any warnings about hypertension. Talk to your doctor about all medications. Never stop taking your antihypertensive medication on your own in order to take another medication. Ask your pharmacist about the effect of a medication on blood pressure when filling a prescription, or buying a nonprescription drug.

> ### That's a Lot of Counters
> There are over 300,000 medications containing 700 active ingredients available "over the counter" (not requiring a prescription).

Let's look at some drugs that may pose problems in hypertension, beginning with oral contraceptives.

Oral contraceptives

Medications that contain estrogen, such as oral contaceptives, can raise the blood pressure. For example, hypertension has been reported to be two to three times more common in women taking the pill for five years or more than in women not taking an oral contraceptive for the same length of time.

Oral contraceptives also increase the risk of a person with hypertension having a stroke. (They also increase the risk for stroke among women who smoke cigarettes.)

So if you are taking an oral contraceptive and develop hypertension, your doctor may insist that you stop the pill.

Be sure to discuss alternative methods of birth control with your doctor if you are taken off an oral contraceptive.

Here are some other drugs that can pose problems with hypertension.

Adrenal steroids

Examples: cortisone, hydrocortisone, prednisone.

Used for: various forms of inflammation and inflammatory-type diseases.

Note: Adrenal steroids are often absolutely necessary to take. They should never be stopped abruptly, and should not even be reduced except under the guidance of a physician.

Antacids (some)

Examples: antacids containing sodium.

Used for: gastritis and stomach and duodenal ulcers.

Check the label or talk to your doctor or pharmacist before taking an antacid.

Antidepressants (some)

Examples: amitriptyline and other tricyclic antidepressants, MAO inhibitors.

Used for: depression.

Note: Certain types of antidepressants, including the newer serotonin antagonists, do not affect blood pressure.

Cocaine

Yes, it is a drug, and hypertension is only one of many reasons to stay away from it.

Cyclosporine

Used for: organ transplant.

Erythropoietin

Used for: certain types of anemia.

NSAIDs (nonsteroidal anti-inflammatory drugs)

Examples: all drugs containing ibuprofen, plus others.

Used for: headache, arthritis, other types of pain and inflammation.

These drugs vary greatly in their effect on BP. Their long-term effects on hypertension are unknown.

Sympathomimetics

Examples: anything containing phenylephrine, ephedrine, pseudoephedrine.

Used for: colds, sinus conditions, allergies, asthma, appetite suppression (diet pills).

A final plea: Rely on the advice of your physician and pharmacist about what to take and what not to take. Always read medication labels carefully—they are there to protect you.

Work

Sometimes medications cause the blood pressure to fall too low, resulting in temporary light-headedness, even blackout. People who operate dangerous equipment, work in high places, and perform any other activity where this could pose a problem need to make their doctor aware of such responsibilities.

Your company clinic should be made aware of the fact that you have hypertension and any medications you are taking.

Stress

We talked about the blood pressure elevation that occurs in "flight or fight" before. It's a normal reaction to stressful circumstances. Since stress is part of our daily living, the best advice is to simply keep your blood pressure under optimal day-to-day control, and the transient rises due to everyday anxieties shouldn't be a problem.

You should also learn and practice your own personal antidotes for stress, such as exercise and other forms of regular relaxation.

Sleep

Lack of sleep, either too few hours or improper quality, causes fatigue. And in some folks fatigue raises the blood pressure.

A problem we don't yet fully understand is called *sleep apnea.* This often occurs in people who snore and have restless sleep. The combination of snoring and restless sleep is associated with high blood pressure, not just at night, but during the day as well.

And it's not as simple as taking a sleeping pill, either. Snoring and restless sleep should be reported to your doctor.

Regular Hours

Your blood pressure is one part of a remarkable, regularly recurring symphony of hormonal changes over each span of twenty-four hours. It's part of the circadian rhythm we discussed earlier.

This makes it desirable to try to live each day according to a regular pattern of activities. To get in concert with your hormones, you should go to sleep, arise, eat, exercise, and take your medications at about the same time each day. If you take your blood pressure, you should take it at set times as your doctor instructs you.

Travel

Modern-day travel is hard on everybody. But high blood pressure isn't a reason to stay at home, unless your doctor doesn't believe that your BP is satisfactorily controlled.

When you do travel, there are a few things you should know.

Standard airline food is second only to Mama Carlone's pizza in its salt content. Fix your own sack lunch or call ahead to the airline—at least twenty-four hours—and order a low-sodium meal. Watch out for restaurant food, too—it can also be very salty.

Take two complete supplies of your blood pressure medicine with you, packed separately, especially if you are going abroad. Medicines dispensed in the United States are not necessarily available in other countries, and when they are, they may be under different names.

Crossing three or more time zones can be rough on the body's clock. Because of the desirability of regular patterns of activity, ask your doctor for advice on how to adjust yourself to a new schedule, and follow it as soon as you arrive.

If you become ill, be certain to tell the doctor caring for you that you have hypertension and what medications you take.

Final Thought

As you can see, there's a lot you can do to help yourself if you have hypertension. If it all seems kind of overwhelming, be assured that it will just take a little time and patience before these new habits become second nature to you.

One more thing. There's very little we've recommended that everyone, even those who think they're in perfect health, shouldn't also follow. And much of it is just common sense, taking you toward a healthier and happier way of living every day, the way your body likes it.

It's Your Turn

1. What is your weight?

_____ pounds

2. What is your ideal weight?*

_____ pounds

3. Calculate the number of pounds you need to lose to achieve your ideal weight is (1 minus 2) _____.

4. Do you smoke?
   ❏ Yes*   ❏ No

5. Do you believe you eat too much salt?
   ❏ Yes*   ❏ No

6. Do you believe you eat too much fat?
   ❏ Yes*   ❏ No

7. Do you believe alcohol might be a factor in your hypertension?
   ❏ Yes*   ❏ No

8. Do you exercise:
   ❏ Regularly
   ❏ Irregularly*
   ❏ Not at all*

9. Based on your answers 1–8, write down what you are going to do for yourself to help lower your blood pressure:

_____

_____

_____

Good for you!

*Discuss this with your doctor if you haven't already done so or you are unsure of the answer.

4

Antihypertensive Medications

The Miracle Drugs

F EW OTHER TYPES of drugs have proven as effective as the modern antihypertensive medications in preventing serious illness. Deaths from coronary heart disease and stroke have fallen more than 50 percent over the past several years, in large part due to better treatment of hypertension.

But, as amazing as these medications are, people taking them should not be lulled into a false sense of security. Blood pressure is only one of several factors contributing to diseases of the heart, kidneys, and blood vessels. Diet, avoiding smoking, proper exercise, weight control, and just common sense about taking proper care of your body become no less important when medications bring down the blood pressure, even to normal levels.

So, no matter how well these drugs take care of your blood pressure, your own lifestyle, which we talked about in chapter 3, remains vitally important.

Goals

The aim of every person with hypertension should be to bring the blood pressure down into the normal range, and keep it there. This includes the very elderly, who clearly benefit from antihypertensive treatment. By *normal range*, we mean a systolic pressure under 140mm Hg, and a diastolic pressure under 90mm Hg. However, for those few who can't get their pressures completely down to normal, *any* reduction is beneficial and well worth the cost and effort.

Blood pressure reduction is carried out in two ways. First, some people whose hypertension isn't too bad can achieve normal blood pressures with lifestyle changes alone, discussed in chapter 3. But for most folks, antihypertensive medications and lifestyle changes are both needed.

Just how far the blood pressure should be lowered below the target goals of under 140mm Hg systolic and under 90mm Hg diastolic is an area of controversy, centered on what researchers call the "J curve." Some research suggests that lowering the diastolic pressure below 85mm Hg with medications might increase the risk for some cardiovascular problems, such as heart attack. This is a special concern in the elderly. Until we learn whether there really is a "J curve" problem, you should have a clear understanding with your doctor about the lower limit on your BP.

Starting Antihypertensive Medications

As you'll soon see, your doctor has a huge selection of antihypertensive medications to choose from. Which of these drugs is used to begin treatment, when it is started, and its dose are determined by a variety of factors, including:

- The stage of hypertension
- The presence of target organ disease
- The presence of other risk factors
- The presence of other conditions or diseases
- Other medications being taken

Other considerations are age and ethnic background. Direct drug costs and secondary costs related to the drug, such as follow-up office visits and tests, also enter into the decision.

When your doctor starts your medical treatment, this is the beginning of a process of trial and error which may extend over several weeks, maybe even months, until the exact regimen that's right for you is found. This is going to establish your therapy for a long time, maybe years, so this period should not be rushed.

Down on the Pharm

"Pharmacy" comes to us from the Greek word *pharmakon,* for drug. Here are some more pharms to add to your vocabulary:

pharmacist—person who puts the pills in the bottle and answers two million questions a day about those pills

pharmacognosy—study of drugs from plants

pharmacokinetics—how drugs move around inside your body

pharmacologist—person who studies drugs

pharmacomania—abnormal desire to take drugs

pharmacophiliac—person who has an abnomal desire to take drugs

pharmacophobia—abnormal fear of drugs

Now you know: your mother-in-law is a pharmacophiliac.

Stage 1 and Stage 2 Hypertension

Many people with Stage 1 and Stage 2 hypertension are treated with only lifestyle modifications for the first three to six months. If the blood pressure stays over 140/90, then a medication will probably be started. However, some doctors prefer not to start a medication for BPs in the 140–149/90–94 range unless other risk factors or target organ disease is present.

Experts agree that *monotherapy*—a single drug—should be used to start treatment. At least half of all patients treated for hypertension can be controlled with monotherapy. Which drug depends on individual considerations. Diuretics, beta-blockers, calcium antagonists, ACE inhibitors, alpha-blockers, and alpha-beta-blockers can all be used in Stages 1 and 2 as the first drug.

Regardless of the drug, the lowest dose will be prescribed at the outset. This dose is continued for at least several weeks. After that time:

- If the BP falls to the target range and side effects are absent or insignificant, then the starting dose is established as the permanent dose.
- If the BP has fallen into the target range, but side effects are significant, then a second drug might be substituted.
- If the BP has not fallen into the target range, then your doctor has three choices: increase the dose; stop the medication and try another; or add a small dose of a second medication—usually a diuretic if this wasn't the first choice.

Notice the emphasis on *small* doses; this is the best way to keep side effects to a minimum.

After the exact medications and their doses are established, it may be possible to switch to one of the combination medications. This has the advantage of simplifying the treatment, although combination drugs may cost more.

Stage 3 and Stage 4 Hypertension

Treatment of these stages differs from treatment of Stages 1 and 2 hypertension in several ways. The approach is more aggressive due to the severity of the hypertension and the increased possibility that target organ damage is already present.

First, your doctor may decide not to have a trial of lifestyle changes alone, but rather *start lifestyle changes and medications at the same time.*

Second, you may be given *two* medications at the outset.

Third, *higher doses* of the drugs are usually required, and the doses may be increased sooner.

Fourth, *stronger types* of medications may be needed.

Fifth, *hospitalization* may be necessary if the BP is very high or if, for some other reason, the treatment carries significant risk.

Maintenance Therapy

After your blood pressure has been brought down to normal, or to the level your doctor has set for you, you enter the maintenance phase. During this time the medications and the doses are kept the same, as long as the BP stays controlled. Your concerns now are continuing your lifestyle changes, careful monitoring to be sure the pressure doesn't start rising or isn't driven too low, and avoiding undesirable drug effects. We'll discuss the maintenance period in detail in chapter 5.

Now take a deep breath, and we'll take a closer look at the miracle drugs.

The Antihypertensive Medications

There are several basic drug types that may be prescribed for hypertension. Each type works differently from the others to lower blood pressure. There are several drugs in each type, usually very similar to one another, but sometimes important differences exist, especially among the calcium antagonists. These drugs are usually given in a pure form, but sometimes two different types (almost always a diuretic plus a drug from one other type) may be mixed in the same tablet or capsule—called a "combination product."

Brand Name vs. Generic

Each drug has two names: a brand or trademark name, the name given by the maker, and a generic name, the general chemical name of the product. For example: *Aldactone* (spironolactone). *Aldactone* is the brand name and spironolactone is the generic name. Pharmaceutical companies hold a patent on a drug for seventeen years. After the patent expires, other companies are free to produce the drug, which is then sold under the generic name and often additional brand names as well.

Diuretics

The diuretics, or "water pills," are the most widely used type of antihypertensive medication, although less so today than in the past. Their effectiveness varies greatly from person to person. Many physicians prefer to use a diuretic as the first drug in treating hypertension. They also work well in combination with the other types of antihypertensive medications when a second drug is added.

How they act

Exactly how diuretics lower the blood pressure isn't certain, but their action clearly relates to their effect on sodium in the body. When you take a diuretic, two things happen that lower the blood pressure:

- First, they act directly on the kidney, causing sodium to be excreted in the urine. The sodium pulls water out of the bloodstream with it. This "shrinks" the volume of blood, lowering the blood pressure.

- Second, the diuretics also appear to act directly on the walls of the small arteries, causing them to dilate and thus lower the blood pressure.

Because the diuretics have a remarkable ability to get rid of unwanted sodium from the body, they are also often used to treat patients with heart failure, as well as other conditions in which excess water is retained in the body.

Pure Forms of Diuretics

Aldactone (spironolactone)
Anhydron (cyclothiazide)
Bumex (bumetanide)
Diucardin (hydroflumethiazide)
Diuril (chlorothiazide)
Dyrenium (triamterene)
Edecrin (ethacrynic acid)
Enduron (methyclothiazide)
Esidrix (hydrochlorothiazide)
Exna (benzthiazide)
HydroDIURIL, Oretic (hydrochlorothiazide)
Hydromox (quinethazone)
Hygroton, Thalitone (chlorthalidone)
Lasix (furosemide)
Lozol (indapamide)
Midamor (amiloride)
Mykrox, Zaroxolyn (metolazone)
Naqua (trichlormethiazide)
Renese (polythiazide)
Saluron (hydroflumethiazide)

Combination Forms

Aldactazide (hydrochlorothiazide + spironolactone)

Dyazide, Maxzide (hydrochlorothiazide + triamterene)

Moduretic (hydrochlorothiazide + amiloride)

Advantages

Diuretics are generally very effective, especially in African-Americans and the elderly.

- They are taken only once a day.
- Because they are prescribed so often, your doctor has a lot of experience with diuretics.
- They are tolerated very well.
- They work well with other antihypertensive drugs when multidrug regimes are necessary.
- They are the least expensive of all antihypertensive medications.

Diuretics are also used to treat heart failure, making them one of the choices when both hypertension and heart failure are present.

Disadvantages

For Stage 3 and Stage 4 hypertension, diuretics by themselves are rarely sufficient.

Even some patients in Stages 1 and 2 do not get enough anti-hypertensive effect when diuretics are used alone.

Diuretics also cause problems with your body's potassium. Depending on which diuretic you take, this can be either a washout of potassium from your body, resulting in dangerously low amounts of potassium, or holding too much potassium in, resulting in dangerously high amounts of potassium circulating in the bloodstream. The combination forms listed above all contain two diuretics, one that tends to cause potassium loss, and another that causes potassium retention; they have been combined in order to balance each other and keep the potassium normal. Even with the combination forms, however, the blood potassium needs to be monitored. (Keeping your potassium at the right level is easy to do, provided you follow your doctor's instructions. Because there are no reliable symptoms of either high or low potassium, this centers on having your blood potassium checked frequently when starting treatment, and on a regular basis after you are stabilized.)

Diuretics have several other effects on the body's metabolism. These include raising the uric acid (sometimes causing gout), blood sugar (worsening the control of diabetes), calcium, total cholesterol, and triglycerides. Your doctor may want to monitor some or all of these.

Diuretics should be used with caution in diabetics, because of their effects on blood sugar and blood fats. See chapter 7 for more information.

Diuretics can drain your body of too much water, causing detion, which can actually lower your blood pressure too much. Excessive thirst, unaccounted weight reduction, headaches, light-headedness, and dizziness are all warning signs of dehydration.

Uncommon problems caused by diuretics are pancreatitis, skin rashes and other forms of allergies, and diminished sexual activity.

All that being said, we must emphasize that the diuretics are very valuable medications for many people with hypertension, and these problems are almost always easily controllable, *with proper monitoring and attention to your doctor's orders.*

Dosing

Most diuretics are taken once a day for hypertension. This should be in the morning, to avoid being kept awake by frequent urination at night.

Very small doses can be surprisingly effective, especially in the elderly, and should be tried first, to avoid some of the unwanted effects listed above.

Peripheral/Sympatholytic Agents: Beta-Blockers

The beta-blockers are widely used not only for hypertension, but also for a variety of other conditions.

How they act

The beta-blockers lower the blood pressure in two ways: They reduce the force of the heartbeat, and they interfere with a potent group of hormones affecting the blood pressure, called the *renin-angiotensin system.*

Beta-Blockers:

Blocadren (timolol)

Cartrol (carteolol)

Corgard (nadolol)

Inderal (propranolol)

Kerlone (betaxolol)

Levatol (penbutolol)

Lopressor, Toprol XL (metoprolol)

Normodyne, *
Trandate*
(labetalol*)

Sectral (acebutolol)

Tenormin (atenolol)

Visken (pindolol)

*These are technically "alpha-beta-blockers," with some differences from pure beta-blockers, such as favorable effect on the blood fats.

Advantages

The beta-blockers are very effective drugs, generally more potent than diuretics in treating hypertension, and well tolerated by many people.

They have been used for many years for several different conditions (migraine, anxiety, glaucoma, and central nervous system tremor), so physicians are generally very experienced in using them.

Among patients who also have coronary heart disease, they provide some protective effect on the heart, and can prevent and treat certain types of fast heart rhythms.

Disadvantages

Suddenly stopping a beta-blocker can be dangerous if there is also a heart condition, such as coronary heart disease, present.

While most people feel fine on beta-blockers, many people become very fatigued, sometimes depressed. Exercise can be difficult.

Sleeping disturbances such as insomnia and wild dreams can occur. They can also impair sexual function.

Excessive fall of the blood pressure in the upright condition, called orthostatic hypotension, may happen. This is more common with the alpha-beta-blockers.

Asthma and other bronchitis-related conditions may become worse. Other conditions that can worsen while on beta-blockers include emphysema, kidney disease, heart failure, heart block, claudication, and diabetes mellitus. *If you have any of these medical conditions, be sure your doctor knows about it before taking a beta-blocker.*

Blood fats can become abnormal, with a rise in the triglycerides and fall of the HDL cholesterol.

Although beta-blockers are often successful in treating hypertension in African-Americans and the elderly, these groups do not respond as well as others.

Dosing

Beta-blockers are taken once or twice (every twelve hours) a day.

Peripheral/Sympatholytic Agents: Alpha-Blockers

How they act

Alpha-blockers interfere with the nerve impulses to the small arteries, causing these vessels to dilate, thereby lowering the blood pressure.

> **Alpha-Blockers:**
>
> *Cardura* (doxazosin)
>
> *Hytrin* (terazosin)
>
> *Minipress* (prazosin)

Advantages

They are not as likely as beta-blockers to worsen certain underlying conditions, such as asthma.

The alpha-blockers are among the few antihypertensive medications to have a favorable effect on blood lipids.

Disadvantages

They may cause an excessive fall in blood pressure in the upright position, occasionally to the point of passing out, *especially with the first dose*. They must therefore be used very cautiously with the elderly.

Headaches, dizziness, dry mouth, fluid retention, drowsiness, and urinary incontinence can occur.

African-Americans do not respond as well to alpha-blockers as to many other antihypertensive medications.

Dosing

Hytrin and *Cardura*—once a day.

Minipress—twice a day.

Peripheral Adrenergic Neuron Antagonists

These drugs can be very difficult to take, due to side effects, and are used mainly for Stage 3 and Stage 4 hypertension.

> **Neuron Antagonists:**
> *Ismelin* (guanethidine); *Hylorel* (guanadrel); *Diupres, Diutensen, Hydropres, Ser-Ap-Es, Regroton, Salutensin* (combinations of reserpine plus diuretics).

How they act

Similar to the alpha-blockers, these drugs also interfere with the nerve impulses to the small arteries, causing these vessels to dilate, lowering the blood pressure.

Advantages

Guanethidine and guanadrel are more potent than the alpha- and beta-blockers, and usually reserved for more severe blood pressure elevations, in which they can be very effective.

They are relatively inexpensive.

Disadvantages

They often cause a marked fall in blood pressure in the upright position and sometimes with exercise.

They may cause fluid retention.

Guanethidine may worsen asthma.

Diarrhea is common.

Reserpine and preparations containing reserpine may cause drowsiness, depression (*may be severe, and has been associated with suicide*), nightmares, nasal stuffiness, and stomach and colon problems.

Dosing

Guanethidine and reserpine—once a day.

Guanadrel—twice a day.

Central Sympatholytic Agents

How they act

These drugs interfere with the nerve impulses sent from the BP control center of the brain to the heart, kidneys, and arteries.

> **Central Sympatholytic Agents:**
> *Aldomet* (methyldopa)
> *Catapres* (clonidine)
> *Tenex* (guanfacine)
> *Wytensin* (guanabenz)

Advantages

These are generally older, "backup" medications when other medications cannot be used, or when additional potency is needed to gain control.

Disadvantages

The central sympatholytic agents often cause considerable drowsiness and fatigue.

Orthostatic hypotension and dry mouth are common.

Intestinal, liver, and blood cell abnormalities can occur with methyldopa.

Dosing

Twice per day, except for the patch form of *clonidine* (weekly) and once per day for guanfacine.

ACE Inhibitors

ACE Inhibitors:
Accupril (quinapril)
Altace (ramipril)
Capoten (captopril)
Lotensin (benazepril)
Monopril (fosinopril)
Prinivil , Zestril
(lisinopril)
Renormax (spirapril)
Vasotec (enalapril)

Although they have been in use for many years, ACE inhibitors are one of the newest types of antihypertensive medications. They have gained widespread popularity because of their effectiveness and much better patient acceptance than the older medications.

How they act

One of the most important ways the body maintains its blood pressure is by means of potent, naturally occurring chemicals in the bloodstream making up what is called the renin-angiotensin (RA) system. Medical scientists have discovered that by preventing the reactions among the RA chemicals from taking place, the blood pressure can be lowered. Substances that do this are called *Angiotensin Converting Enzyme* (ACE) inhibitors.

Advantages

The ACE inhibitors provide remarkable potency and are relatively free of unwanted effects on the body such as postural hypotension, sexual dysfunction, blood sugar elevation, and blood fat abnormalities, which are common to many other antihypertensive medications.

They are also an extremely effective treatment for heart failure.

Disadvantages

The most dangerous problem, although uncommon, is angioedema, which is manifest as acute swelling of the face, tongue, lips, vocal cords, and extremities. *Because this can be life threatening, medical help should be sought immediately, and the drug not taken again unless approved by a physician.*

ACE inhibitors should not be taken by pregnant women, because they can be harmful, even fatal, to the unborn baby.

ACE inhibitors should be avoided in the presence of some forms of lung and kidney disease.

Cough is the main side effect of ACE inhibitors, sometimes bothersome enough to force discontinuation. This can result in an expensive diagnostic evaluation for other causes of cough, since it cannot always be assumed a cough is due to the medication.

Loss of taste and appetite are common.

As with all antihypertensives, the blood pressure can fall too low, especially if taken with a diuretic.

Elevated blood potassium levels can occur if a potassium-sparing diuretic or potassium supplements are taken with an ACE inhibitor.

African-Americans do not respond as well to ACE inhibitors as other populations do.

Dosing

ACE inhibitors can usually be taken once per day, but sometimes twice per day is necessary for optimal blood pressure control.

Calcium Antagonists

Calcium Antagonists:
Calan, *Verelan*
  (verapamil)
Cardene (nicardipine)
Cardizem, Dilacor
  (diltiazem)
DynaCirc (isradipine)
Norvasc (amlodipine)
Plendil (felodipine)
Procardia (nifedipine)

This is another relatively new type of antihypertensive medication that has gained widespread use in recent years as a result of its potency and good patient acceptance. Some of these drugs work well in the face of continued high salt intake. They are also a highly effective treatment for coronary heart disease and have been used in treating migraine.

How they act

Calcium antagonists influence the flow of calcium in and out of cells, including the cells of blood vessels, causing the small arteries to dilate, reducing the pressure. It should be emphasized that these drugs have *nothing* to do with the amount of calcium in the diet, or the blood calcium level.

Advantages

These drugs are very potent and well tolerated by most people.

They do not affect the body's lipids or glucose and don't cause postural hypotension.

They are also used to treat angina pectoris in patients with coronary heart disease, and to control certain heart-rhythm disturbances.

African-Americans tend to respond better to these drugs than to ACE inhibitors and to beta-blockers.

Disadvantages

Dizziness, constipation, headache, edema (swelling in the lower extremities), and swollen gums can occur.

Verapamil and diltiazem preparations can cause heart block and heart failure. Other calcium antagonists can cause a rapid heartbeat and flushing.

Dosing

One to three times per day, depending on the drug.

Direct Vasodilators

How they act

The vasodilators act directly on the arteries, causing them to enlarge, lowering the pressure.

Direct Vasodilators:
Apresoline (hydralazine)
Loniten, others (minoxidil)

Advantages

They are very potent, especially minoxidil, making them useful in advanced stages of hypertension.

Disadvantages

Because they frequently cause a fast heartbeat and water retention, they generally must be given with other antihypertensives, which counteract these effects.

Hydralazine sometimes causes an illness called lupus, with rash and arthritis. Vasodilators can also cause GI disturbances, headache, dizziness, and nasal congestion.

Minoxidil causes excessive hair growth and fluid retention.

Dosing

Hydralazine: two to four times per day.
Minoxidil: one to two times per day.

Whew!

Gives you some idea why medical school takes so long, doesn't it?

Obviously, your doctor has plenty of medications to choose from. However, except for specialists who work exclusively with hypertension patients, no physician has a working knowledge of *all* medications. Fortunately, one or two drugs of each type are all your doctor really needs to know in detail.

Rules to Live By

Regardless of what drug or combination of drugs you need to control your blood pressure, there are some important general guidelines for you to follow, for optimal control and safety.

1. Except for an obvious adverse reaction, *never discontinue medications on your own.* When a reaction does occur, consult your physician immediately.

2. *Don't discontinue your medications because your blood pressure falls and stays normal,* either—it just means the drug, or drugs, are doing their job.

3. *Never increase or decrease the drug doses on your own.* For example, some folks have been known to get a headache or some other side effect, and conclude that their blood pressure must be up and then take an extra dose of their antihy-

pertensive medication. Never, ever, do this. Remember, how you feel is not a reliable reflection of your blood pressure, and changing doses of medications on your own is dangerous.

4. *Take your medications at the same time each day*. Your blood pressure has a regular pattern of rises and falls throughout the day and night (the circadian rhythm again), and it's best if your medication can become part of that pattern. It's also a lot easier to remember to take your medications if taken on a fixed schedule.

5. *Know your medication*. After all, it has become part of your body's everyday chemistry. Its side effects, hazards, the correct way to take it, and cross-reactions with other drugs are all important for you to know. Read the information that comes with the drug, and ask your pharmacist and physician if they have any additional material about the drug.

6. *Ask your doctor or pharmacist before you take other medications*, either nonprescription or prescription. They could interfere with your blood pressure control. For example, NSAIDs, which are popular drugs for pain, may reduce the effectiveness of your antihypertensive medication.

7. *Attention to lifestyle* remains important—for the rest of your life, even when you take "miracle" drugs.

How Long?

Hypertension is a lifelong illness requiring lifelong treatment. This usually means medications for the rest of your life.

A Final Plea

Know what the single biggest problem with treating hypertension is?

Taking the antihypertensive medication as prescribed. Millions of folks don't! It's called *noncompliance,* and it happens for a lot of reasons.

Whatever the reason, if you ever find yourself not taking your medication, talk to your doctor about it. Noncompliance isn't a sin—just something you need to work out. While you still have time.

It's Your Turn

1. List the medications you are taking for your blood pressure:

Brand name	Generic name	Dose
_____	_____	_____
_____	_____	_____
_____	_____	_____

2. List any side effects you are having, or believe you are having from these medications:

_____ *

_____ *

_____ *

3. Do you take any other medications for other reasons, either prescription or nonprescription?

❑ Yes*   ❑ No

List: _____

4. Do any of the medications you listed in 3 affect the BP or the action of your prescription medications?

❑ Yes*   ❑ No

List: _____

5. The way you take your BP medications is generally:

❑ Very regular, seldom missing a dose

❑ Very irregular, often missing doses*

6. If you answered "very irregular, often missing doses," state the reason:

❏ Can't remember to take them*

❏ Side effects*

❏ Cost*

❏ Other* give:_____

*Talk to your doctor if you haven't already done so, or you are unsure of the answer.

5

How Are You Doing?

YOU RAN YOUR first marathon last weekend—or maybe walked a mile at a brisk pace. . . . You haven't had any gin in your tonic for three months. . . . Your body has become so trim that someone actually pinched you on the elevator—and at your age it'd be a stretch to call it harassment. . . . You burned Mama Carlone's Frozen Pizza box in effigy. . . . Dr. Rex took your BP just before excavating five root canals and it was normal. . . .

As the morning sun brightly illuminates your bedroom, you lie there thinking, "It's a new day, another day to enjoy." You leap out of bed, and the next thing you are aware of is a knot on your forehead as you sprawl facedown on the floor.

Maybe you won't enjoy today as much as you hoped.

What's Going On?

Despite your great strides in adopting a wonderful lifestyle, and the amazing effects of modern antihypertensive medications, you need to remain on guard.

For example, those miracle drugs bring with them their own set of problems. That's why you're lying on the floor. You just experienced *postural hypotension*, just one reason why you need to watch yourself.

There are a lot more reasons, so read on.

New Goals

After your blood pressure was brought down to the level your doctor decided was just right for you, you began a new phase in your life with hypertension, the *maintenance phase*. This is the time for forgetting about hypertension *without really forgetting about it*. Put another way, it means making the control of your hypertension just another aspect of your everyday life. Not a chore, a burden, or a worry. Just one of a hundred other routines you practice every day.

You have three goals for the maintenance phase:

- First, to maintain a normal, or ideal, blood pressure.
- Second, to do whatever else is needed for preventing target organ damage.
- Third, to feel good in the process.

Let's Thank the Vets

The proof that treating hypertension prevented complications didn't come until a historic report in 1967 in the *Journal of the American Medical Association* on a study conducted in conjunction with the Veterans Administration. Using the drugs reserpine, a diuretic, and hydralazine, this study showed that treating hypertension reduced the risk of a serious cardiovascular problem from over 50% to under 20% over a period of five years. Since that historic article there have been many more reports from the United States and other countries showing the value of antihypertensive treatment. But the vets were the first.

The key is to establish, along with all those healthy new activities in your life, a *regular pattern of monitoring yourself*. The way you monitor is threefold: take your blood pressure (or have someone else take it); pay attention to the way you feel; and see your doctor on a regular basis.

Taking Your Blood Pressure

Most doctors and patients find that home blood pressure measurement is very valuable. So do the American Heart Association, the National High Blood Pressure Education Program, and the American Society of Hypertension, *as long as its purpose isn't to self-prescribe and self-diagnose.* However, we're all different, and maybe you'd rather not take your own pressure. Or maybe that's the way your doctor feels. The two of you should talk over its pros and cons.

If you take your own blood pressure, it is absolutely essential you do it correctly. Incorrect blood pressure measurements are worse than none at all, because your doctor will probably use your measurements as one of the guides in prescribing your treatment.

The keys to correctly measuring blood pres-

Sphygmomanometer: From the Greek (those Greeks loved medicine, didn't they?) word *sphygmic,* which relates to the pulse. This is the official name of the instrument used to take the BP. For obvious reasons, we'll just call it a BP monitor.

sure are (1) selecting the appropriate blood pressure monitor (sphygmomanometer) for you; (2) using the proper technique; (3) taking the blood pressure at the right time; and (4) maintaining the accuracy of the blood pressure monitor.

Selecting the Blood Pressure Monitor

There are three basic types of devices for measuring the blood pressure: the mercury manometer, the mechanical aneroid manometer, and the electronic aneroid manometer (finger and arm models).

All three of these devices vary in cost and accuracy. However, the mechanical aneroid type, which is the most compact and least expensive, is suitable if kept calibrated and in good condition. The mercury type, which is most often used in doctors' offices, is the most accurate, but is heavy and bulky. The electronic type can be expensive, is sometimes very inaccurate, and is worthwhile mainly for users who have trouble with a stethoscope.

You might also be tempted to stick your arm or thumb into a coin-operated device next to the candy machine. For a few quarters, it'll give you some numbers that may or may not be close to your real blood pressure. Your money would be better spent on the candy bar (low fat, of course).

AAMI

Your favorite charity, the Association for the Advancement of Medical Instrumentation, has set standards for blood pressure monitors. Manufacturers don't have to comply, but we suggest you don't buy a device unless the package states it meets AAMI's standards.

The Right Technique

The blood pressure monitor comes in a kit, complete with instructions (don't buy it if it doesn't), inflatable cuffs (in various sizes, for big and little arms), a stethoscope (or microphone for electronic devices), and manometer (dial).

We're going to tell you how to do it, but you should still have a "pro" in your doctor's office check out your technique, once you think you've mastered it. They will even be happy to teach you how, just in case we totally confuse you.

Here goes, for a mechanical BP monitor:

1. Sit in a comfortable chair for a few minutes, your arm resting on a table at about the height of your midchest.

2. Place the stethoscope around your neck.

3. Wrap the cuff snugly and evenly around your arm, above the elbow so that the skin doesn't get pinched when the arm is bent.

> **Problem:** The cuff doesn't encircle the arm, meaning its length is too short. **Solution:** Get a longer cuff. It should nearly or completely encircle the arm, or the pressure may be falsely high. Cuff width is important, too, and should be at least 40% of the arm circumference.

4. Feel for the pulsation of your brachial artery, with the forefinger and index finger on the inside front of the elbow, just around the corner from your "funny bone."

> **Problem:** You can't find the pulse. **Solution:** You're either palpating too hard or too softly, or you have a weird brachial artery that isn't where it should be. Try palpating with different degrees of pressure, over the inner half of the front of your elbow.

5. The cuff should have an arrow marked "artery." Position the cuff so that the arrow points to the brachial artery.

> **Problem:** There's no arrow.
> **Solution:** Consider seeking a refund.

6. Place the stethoscope bell, firmly but not hard, over the brachial artery.

7. Place the stethoscope earpieces into your ears, not too tightly.

8. While watching the gauge, pump up the cuff to a point well above (30–60mm Hg) what you know to be your systolic pressure.

There should be no pulsations apparent on the gauge at this point.

9. Slowly release air from the cuff, about 2–3mm Hg per second, while watching the gauge and listening through the stethoscope. At first you shouldn't hear anything. Suddenly, you'll hear a "tapping" sound with each pulsation, and the needle on the gauge (or mercury in the column) will move slightly as well. Note the number on the gauge when the tapping started.

Congratulations! You just found the systolic pressure!

Problem: You don't hear anything. **Possible solutions:** (**1**) Loosen the earpieces—they may be too tight in your ears; (**2**) make sure the stethoscope bell is directly over the brachial artery, and is making total contact with the skin; (**3**) get your hearing tested.

10. Continue releasing air from the cuff. The tapping becomes more of a swishing sound as you do this. Then, as you approach your diastolic pressure, the sound fades gradually, or disappears abruptly. *Careful now, this is tricky.* When the sound *totally* disappears, note the number on the gauge.

Voilà ! This is the diastolic pressure!

Problem: The sound fades, but never totally disappears. (Nothing is wrong; this just happens in some people. Medical students struggle with this, too.) **Solution:** Record the diastolic pressure as the pressure *when the sound makes a definite fade,* even though it never totally disappears. And make note of this fact on your BP record.

11. Repeat the measurement once or twice more, until the numbers are pretty much consistent.

Problem: The numbers never get consistent, and your arm starts to turn an ugly purple from repeatedly pumping up the cuff. **Solution:** Have your technique and the BP monitor checked by your doctor. You should also check your pulse, to be sure it's regular, because an irregular heart rhythm can cause wide variations in the blood pressure.

12. Record all the numbers. If you're mathematically inclined, average them.

You've done it!

This Is Embarrassing

Doctors don't always do it right, either. A few years ago over a hundred doctors were watched for their technique when taking blood pressures. Here's how they did:

96% didn't allow a resting period.

77% didn't measure in both arms.

90% didn't compare sitting and standing pressures.

97% used the wrong size cuff.

82% didn't deflate the cuff at the right rate.

Something to remember when you get the bill.

The Right Time

This is crucial.

Your blood pressure, whether normal or totally out of control, shows huge changes depending on the time of day (remember the circadian rhythm?). Physical activity, your mental state, and the time you took your last dose of medication all greatly influence the blood pressure. So your blood pressure reading really has a lot less meaning unless these are taken into account.

There are basically two times for taking the blood pressure. One is the *baseline reading,* and the other is a *random reading.*

The baseline reading should be made at a specific time of day. Other activities should be consistent on the days such readings are taken, including the length of time since awakening from sleep, meals, exercise, and last dose of medication. You should not use tobacco or drink caffeinated beverages within an hour before measuring your blood pressure. One of the best times is right before you take a dose of the antihypertensive medication. Another good time is a certain number of hours after you take the medication, particularly during its peak effect (your doctor can tell you when). Baseline readings may be daily, weekly, or at whatever frequency your doctor wants. Don't be neurotic about it, just *consistent*.

Random readings are more difficult to interpret, and are designed to determine how your blood pressure is responding to various circumstances and various symptoms, such as finding yourself face down with your nose buried in the carpet.

The main thing is to be sure to record the time of day, exact circumstances, and how you felt at the time. Don't trust your memory.

Both baseline and random readings, times, and special notations should be kept in a single notebook, small enough to be carried with you. Always take the book with you when you visit the doctor, who'll love you for it.

Maintaining the Accuracy

Ever compare your watch with the time on television? Even a Rolex ought to be checked now and then.

You need to calibrate your blood pressure monitor at least once a year, too. Not with the television set, of course, but with your doctor's office sphygmomanometer. Have them check your BP on both their mercury manometer and your device at the same time. If the readings aren't the same, then make the correction as outlined on the instructions that came with your monitor. If you can't do that, then you should make a mathematical correction each time you take your blood pressure at home.

A few other points about accuracy. If you have an aneroid manometer, the needle should point to zero when the cuff is not inflated. The deflation valve should be able to hold a pressure above

And the Problem Is . . .
What goes wrong with BP monitors? Here are some leading problems:

• faulty control valve

• gauge not on zero when cuff deflated

• cracked face plate

• bad rubber tubing

your systolic pressure until released. And after release, you should be able to control deflation to fall no faster than 3mm/sec.

Feeling Good

You probably felt fine before you discovered you had hypertension. You *still* should feel good, maybe even better if you've lost some weight and are getting some exercise.

But there are a few things about hypertension that could, if we let them, make life less than you desire. Of course, we're not going to let that happen.

Medications

We sometimes forget that when we take medications, they go to every part of the body, not just where they do some good. Take an aspirin for a headache. It doesn't go just to the head to cure the headache. It also goes to the toes, as well, where it can start an attack of gout.

Antihypertensive drugs are no different. Part of that little pill goes where we want, to the blood vessels, heart, and kidneys to control the blood pressure. But some of it also goes to the lungs, where beta-blockers can precipitate a bout of asthma. And to the skin, where diuretics may cause a rash. And to the face and mouth, where ACE inhibitors sometimes cause swelling.

So undesirable, even dangerous things can happen when you take your antihypertensive medicine. That's why you should be aware of the side effects and precautions of these and every other medicine you take. We mentioned a few of the problems with antihypertensive medications in chapter 4, but we only scratched the surface. You should thoroughly read any written material that comes with the medication, and even ask your doctor or pharmacist for more information. And if you suspect any side effects, even if not listed, tell your doctor *immediately.*

Another reality about antihypertensive drugs is that they are *very potent.* After all, they are acting directly on one of the body's most complex chemical regulatory systems. Ultimately this means affecting the blood flow and metabolism of every living cell in your body!

Although most problems surface soon after a medication is begun, many undesirable effects, both minor and serious, can appear at any time. So a rash, a wheeze, or a swollen joint caused by a medication can occur one hour, one day, or one year after you started taking the drug. Of course, a rash, a wheeze, or a swollen joint aren't necessarily caused by the drug you are taking to lower your blood pressure, either. New problems may be totally unrelated to your blood pressure or drugs you're taking to lower the blood pressure.

Postural Hypotension

Postural hypotension is a common problem caused by many of the antihypertensive medications (some drugs are much more likely to be a cause than others), and is worth special mention. This side effect explains why you landed on the floor this morning when you got out of bed. As the name itself suggests, this is a condition in which the blood pressure falls too far and too fast when changing from a reclining or sitting position to standing.

Think about our friends at the waterworks again. What if your house were suddenly lifted several stories up in the air by a great underground swelling? If you were taking a shower at that moment, you would have a hard time rinsing the soap off, as the water pressure would quickly fall to zero.

Now compare your head to your house. When your head suddenly goes from a "down" position, like on the pillow, to five or six feet above the floor, your cardiovascular system must undergo drastic circulatory changes to maintain the blood pressure in your head. Normally, such a postural change is something the body handles with incredible efficiency, unlike the city waterworks.

But some antihypertensive medications block your body's ability to maintain the blood pressure when you change position. The result can be a fall in the pressure for several seconds, long enough for you to become dizzy or even lose consciousness. And you end up smelling the carpet.

Postural hypotension is a frequent problem in the elderly. And it's a special threat to older folks with osteoporosis, which can lead to a hip fracture with even a small fall. Postural hypotension is also more common in people with diabetes mellitus.

What do you do about postural hypotension? Most important, *tell your doctor right away* if you fall when you stand up, or even if you get light-headed, especially if you are elderly. Your doctor *(not you*) may need to adjust your antihypertensive medication, which may be a simple matter of changing the dose. One way to find out whether you have postural hypotension, if it can't be proven in the doctor's office, is to take your own blood pressure both sitting and standing at various times of the day, particularly at the time of peak action of the antihypertensive medication.

There are lots of other causes of temporary unconsciousness. These include transient ischemic attacks (TIAs, or "small strokes"), heart block, low blood sugar, loss of blood, even severe dehydration. So landing on the floor isn't *necessarily* caused by the antihypertensive medication.

Additional caution: Until your doctor determines the exact cause and treatment of these spells, and they are corrected, it is very important not to operate vehicles and other hazardous equipment.

A final note about undesirable effects caused by antihypertensives: You don't have to endure them. As we've said, your doctor has plenty of alternative medications to choose from (doctors like to call this their *armamentarium*, their weapons arsenal against hypertension). Somewhere out there, in that vast pharmaceutical universe, is the combination of drugs and doses that's just right for you.

Despite how good they ultimately should make you feel overall, lifestyle changes themselves aren't necessarily a joyride, either.

So You Hate Steamed Vegetables

Like diet. On a crash diet and feeling terrible? Having dreams about wolfin' down a chocolate pie?

Whoa.

First, let's take weight loss. No one told you to lose thirty pounds in a month. This isn't an emergency. You've had hypertension for quite a while, and you have a long life in front of you. Weight loss should be gradual, steady. A pound a week is pretty good for most people. Besides, any faster, and you increase the chances of someday gaining it back.

What about salt and fat? In all truth, an occasional Whammyburger, like when you go out to eat with the kids, isn't going to blow your head off on the spot. If you enjoy such strays into the fast-food lanes now and then (and who doesn't?), then go ahead, enjoy them. Just do it in moderation, like rewarding yourself with a hamburger on the weekend, or, god forbid, even a sliver or two of Mama Carlone's pepperoni. These will be forgiven by your body by eating less salt and fat for the next day or so to make up for that glorious moment of pleasure.

Besides, who knows? After you've been away from salt for a while, maybe you'll discover Mama Carlone didn't make such terrific pizza after all.

Before we leave the subject of diet, we have to add one more comment. The diet you are on isn't really a *diet* at all. Don't look at it like the penalty you have to pay for having hypertension.

This is the way everyone should eat, even if they don't have hypertension.

Jogging, Too

- How are you doing with your exercise?
- If you say thirty to forty-five minutes, a few days a week, good.
- If you say two hours a week, only on Saturdays, bad.
- If you walk some days and swim others, with a day in the garden now and then, excellent.
- If you're up to four hundred pounds pressing barbells, that's not what we—or your doctor—had in mind.
- If you look forward to whatever you do—except the barbells—terrific.
- If you dread the morning walk, try the evening.

Like your eating habits, exercise should be simply a part of your daily routine, not something special you have to do just because you have hypertension. Be positive; this is that one time of the day for you to take care of yourself, to relax, to reflect, to take in the outdoors, to feel good about your world.

And also like your new way of eating, regular exercise is what you should be doing anyway.

Bah Humbug

How are you doing mentally? Maybe a little tendency to get depressed? Or maybe *very* depressed a lot of the time since learning you have hypertension?

Depression is a common reaction to learning of any chronic illness, especially one that we might *mistakenly* blame on aging. A disease that also carries the threat of heart attack and stroke. And one that we are constantly reminding ourselves about, by taking blood pressures, shunning our beloved pizza, and swallowing strange-sounding medications.

They All Can Do It
All types of antihypertensive medications (even drugs used as placebos in research of hypertension!) can affect the way we "mentally" feel. This includes dizziness, drowsiness, sedation, fatigue, somnolence, insomnia, confusion, depression, and tiredness. But you don't have to feel this way, and some drugs are much more likely to cause these symptoms than others. Talk to your doctor about them if they occur.

So it's understandable, but not necessary, that you might be depressed.

Here are some ways to help you cope with the depression.

First, talk to your doctor about it. *It's possible your medication could be causing the depression.* This is a common side effect of reserpine and also can occur with the beta-blocker medications. For this reason, these drugs sometimes have to be given in lower doses or even stopped altogether.

Second, let's face the way you really feel about having hypertension. This fact doesn't depress most people, but, of course, you are not most people. You are *you.* If you are a little glum about having hypertension, don't keep your feelings to yourself. Have a heart-to-heart talk with your spouse, or a friend, or somebody who cares about you personally. Not for their advice, but for their ears. It's amazing how talking about something like hypertension can make you feel better.

Finally, depression sometimes just doesn't respond to reason. That's because depression is associated with chemical changes in the brain. If you are too depressed, your doctor may want you to take a medication called an antidepressant. This may be for only a short period of time, like a few months, until things are back on track. Talk to your doctor about it. Caution: Remember, certain older antidepressants, called MAO inhibitors and tricyclics, may worsen hypertension.

Sex

Sex can become a problem in hypertension for a variety of reasons.

First, there are the medications themselves. Many of them can either reduce libido or create impotence. Much of this has to do with the drugs' interference with the function of the sympathetic nervous system, which is important to sexual performance, especially in men. But it would be a mistake to automatically assume a drug is the culprit. Your doctor can quickly tell whether your medication should be suspect.

Second, there is the emotional reaction to having hypertension, mostly *fear*. Sometimes folks are anxious about sex because, "as everyone knows," it raises the blood pressure. If your routine blood pressures are controlled, then the blood pressure elevation that normally goes with sex should be no problem.

Third, there is the chance that an associated, possibly hidden disease, such as diabetes or atherosclerosis, can be interfering with sexual performance. Another reason to talk to your doctor.

Preventing Organ Damage

The main reason for treating hypertension is to prevent damage to vital organs and blood vessels. With this in mind, remember that controlling the blood pressure is only part of the task. How well you are preventing target organ damage is an important reason for seeing your doctor regularly, in addition to having your blood pressure checked. Evidence of new organ damage tells your doctor to be more aggressive in treatment of the blood pressure, whether that means increasing the dose of your antihypertensive medications or even changing medications.

Like hypertension itself, organ

For Better or for Worse
Certain antihypertensive medications may—but not always—affect other risk factors and diseases. Here's how (positive = possible favorable effect; negative = possible unfavorable effect):

Blood lipids
    Alpha-blockers—positive
    Beta-blockers—negative
    Diuretics—negative
Gout
    ACE inhibitors—positive
    Diuretics—negative
Diabetes mellitus
    ACE inhibitors—positive
    Alpha-blockers—positive
    Beta- blockers—negative
    Diuretics—negative
Heart failure
    ACE inhibitors—positive
    Alpha-blockers—positive
    Beta-blockers—negative
    Diuretics—positive

damage tends to be a "silent" process, meaning that how you feel is unreliable for detecting metabolic, blood vessel, heart, and kidney abnormalities. Repeat physical checks, blood tests (especially for cholesterol and other blood fats), and other tests, such as electrocardiograms, are often necessary. They can be compared for changes with the results obtained during earlier evaluations.

Exactly what tests, and when they are performed, is highly variable, depending on previous results, your age, the severity of the hypertension, and other factors.

The main thing is this: While the number one goal is to bring your blood pressure down and keep it down, the blood pressure is only one of several risk factors you need to pay attention to.

Why Isn't It Coming Down?
(Or Why Didn't It Stay Down?)

So you've started on antihypertensive medications and changed your lifestyle. The blood pressure's come down—*some*—but not to normal. Or perhaps your blood pressure came down for a while, then went back up.

What's going on?

You may have *resistant hypertension.* If so, here's a checklist of questions to consider:

• *Are you taking your medications exactly as prescribed?* If not, it isn't a sin, but something doesn't have to be a sin to kill you. Of course, doctors' term for it, "noncompliance," makes it sound like a sin. Fact is, it's hard for everyone—including your doctor—to take even a single pill every day, unless that pill is making you feel better, which antihypertensives seldom do. That's why half of all instances of so-called refractory hypertension occur because the drug isn't being taken properly, if at all.

What you can do about noncompliance is first and foremost, *without guilt*, talk to your

Things that May Elevate the BP

• Alcohol
• Amphetamines
• Anabolic (body-builder's) steroids
• Caffeine
• Chlorpromazine
• Cocaine
• Corticosteroids
• Cyclosporine
• Erythropoietin
• Monamine oxidase inhibitors (MAO inhibitors)
• Nicotine
• NSAID
• Oral contraceptives
• Shock-wave lithotripsy
• Sodium chloride (salt pills)
• Sympathomimetic agents (cold, allergy, asthma preparations)
• Tricyclic antidepressants

doctor about it. The solution could be something as simple as keeping a daily drug diary—which isn't a bad idea anyway. Or perhaps changing the time you take it, such as attaching it to some regular event, like part of your breakfast. Or, if you sometimes just don't have the money in the bank to buy the drug, your doctor will have suggestions to take care of that, too. Whatever the problem, your doctor's heard it before, and will be able to help.

- *Are you taking another treatment that interferes with your medication, or raises the blood pressure?* We talked about this in chapter 2.
- *Is there something wrong with your metabolism that elevates the blood pressure?* Obesity and diabetes can make treatment more difficult.
- *Is there another disease raising the BP?* We covered some of these diseases in chapter 2, when we discussed "secondary hypertension."

What If Your Blood Pressure Suddenly Goes Up?

If your BP does rise unexpectedly, it can lead to a *hypertensive emergency* if it goes high enough. As the term implies, this can be very dangerous.

The first sign that you could be headed for a hypertensive emergency is a sudden rise in the blood pressure. You may even have *nonspecific* symptoms, like headache or fatigue. Or you could have *specific* symptoms if one of your organs is in jeopardy, like chest pain from your heart, abdominal pain with an aortic aneurysm, severe headache with bleeding around the brain, and shortness of breath with heart failure.

You never want your blood pressure to rise to the level of causing symptoms. This is one reason why it's important to keep track of your BP *every day.*

When the blood pressure rises suddenly to very high levels, it may be necessary to bring it down quickly. Sometimes, if the pressure is high enough, has risen very rapidly, or target organ damage occurs, hospitalization is required.

What If Your Blood Pressure Is Controlled?

So you've been a model patient for quite a while. Your BP has gone down and it's staying down. What's next? Do you still have to stay on your treatment schedule?

Yes. Absolutely. Now that you've gotten the disease under control, there's no reason to risk bringing it back. You're doing great. Keep it up.

Here's some other encouraging news, at the risk of falsely getting your hopes up. If you've effectively controlled your blood pressure for a year or more, and if you meet certain of your doctor's criteria, it may be possible to reduce the amount of medication you take, *under your doctor's guidance and if you keep following a healthy lifestyle.*

This is called *step-down therapy.* If you qualify for step-down therapy, your doctor will gradually reduce the amount of medication you take. This, of course, is done under close monitoring, and according to a schedule carefully designed by your doctor. At some point, a dose may be reached in response to which the blood pressure starts to go back up. That's when the step-down has to be abandoned. However, it's also possible (but very unlikely) that all drugs can be discontinued entirely without the blood pressure going back up. If this happens, the important thing to remember is that you really aren't cured of hypertension, and constant BP monitoring must continue. Many people eventually see their BPs go back up, and need to return to medications.

It's Your Turn

1. Do you take your own BP?

   ❑ Yes ❑ No

2. If you answered "no" to question 1, have you discussed this possibility with your doctor?

   ❑ Yes ❑ No*

3. When do you take your BP?
   ❑ Randomly, with no definite schedule*
   ❑ Fixed schedule
   ❑ Fixed schedule plus random readings at times

4. At what time of day do your medications have their maximum effect? _____

5. Do you take your BP at this time?
   ❑ Yes   ❑ No

6. If you answered "yes" to question 5, what is your usual BP at this time? _____

7. Do you have symptoms of postural hypotension?
   ❑ Yes*   ❑ No

*Discuss this with your doctor if you haven't already done so or you are unsure of the answer.

6

What Can You Do to Help Control the Cost?

EVERYONE KNOWS health care can be very expensive. But there are different ways to look at it.

In one way, staying healthy is like everything else: We often spend more money on it than is necessary.

On the other hand, our health is *different* from everything else. After all, we've been talking about heart attacks and strokes here, haven't we? That's why it's really easy to adopt a "money is no object" attitude. The problem is, there isn't an infinite supply of money, even for our health.

So what's the answer? It's not easy, but you have already made a great start when you decided to learn as much as you could about hypertension. The more you understand—and act on your understanding—about drugs, diet, tests, taking your own blood pressure, and everything else we've discussed about hypertension, the less expensive it will be.

Being informed is the only certain way to help avoid unnecessary costs, without compromising your health.

Reducing the Pounds

It might be argued that hypertension wouldn't cost any money at all if we didn't treat it. But of course that isn't true. A study conducted in Great Britain a few years ago concluded that for every pound (British, not fat) spent to treat hypertension, three pounds were saved on the cost of caring for strokes that were prevented. This analysis didn't even take heart and kidney disease into account. So, if you want to reduce the whole matter to only dollars and pounds (and we don't), treatment of hypertension still makes sense.

Drugs

As we discussed in chapter 4, there is a huge variety of antihypertensive medications your doctor can choose from. Their costs range from pennies to dollars per day. *Antihypertensive medications account for 70 to 80 percent of total hypertension treatment costs.* Which brings us to a dilemma. The older drugs, like most diuretics, methyldopa, and hydralazine are inexpensive, and newer medications, such as the nongeneric forms of ACE inhibitors and calcium channel blockers, generally cost quite a bit more.

What about generic substitution? This offers considerable savings, provided generic versions of the drug your doctor selected for you are available. However, many excellent, newer medications are not available in generic form. This is a discussion you need to have with your physician. Your pharmacist might be able to help, too.

Why not just ask your doctor to prescribe the older drugs, as long as they bring down the blood pressure and save money? But do they *really* save money? Not necessarily. Older drugs may require closer monitoring—more doctor's visits and tests. For example, if you take a diuretic, you will need to have your blood potassium, blood fats, blood sugar, and uric acid checked from time to time. And if your potassium falls too low, which often happens with diuretics, you may need to add a potassium supplement if dietary supplementation is inadequate.

Another factor is drug side effects. Take the drug hydralazine, for example. While relatively inexpensive, and very effective in lowering the blood pressure, hydralazine commonly causes palpitations and hot, uncomfortable flushing symptoms. In addition, hydralazine sometimes causes an arthritic condition. These problems can result in more visits to the doctor, more tests, and maybe even another medication to counter the side effects of the hydralazine. Another costly alternative is to start over with another antihypertensive medication.

Unfortunately, all medications, old and new, have potential hidden costs associated with them. If these start to occur, you need to talk to your doctor about them.

Another consideration is the dosage. Your doctor will control your blood pressure on the lowest possible dose, mainly for reasons of safety and fewer side effects. But taking the lowest effective dose will also help avoid an unnecessary additional cost. Which brings us to something *you* can do to help costs. Remember, lifestyle changes can have a marked effect on the doses of medications required, and even on whether you need to take *any* medication. Lose weight, restrict salt, exercise, and maybe, just maybe, save some money!

Another possibility for saving money on drugs rests with the

Hidden Costs:

Here are some *potential* problems that might make these drugs more costly than the price tag at the pharmacy:

Diuretics
- lab tests for potassium and other metabolic effects
- potassium and magnesium supplements
- potassium-sparing drugs
- added drugs to lower the blood sugar, uric acid, and blood fats
- added drugs to combat impotence

Beta-blockers
- added antidepressant drugs
- vasodilators
- added drugs to lower blood fats
- added drugs to combat impotence
- added drugs to combat sleep disturbances

ACE inhibitors
- tests for cause of cough
- cough medications
- added drugs to combat itching
- tests to monitor blood count and kidney function

Calcium blockers
- added drugs for headache
- added drugs for constipation
- added drugs for edema
- EKGs to monitor effect on heart

fact that, unlike an antibiotic taken for a week or ten days, you're going to be taking antihypertensive medications for a long time. This makes it possible to get discounts for "bulk purchases," which can be arranged with some pharmacies. Before you buy a thousand water pills, of course, you need to be reasonably certain that they are going to be *your* medication. You should tell your doctor before you do this, just to be sure.

Another way to reduce drug cost is to ask your physician to pre-scribe the medication in amounts double your dose, if it comes in the form of a scored tablet. Then break the tablet in half for your daily dose. This can save as much as 25 percent per dose. Caution: Be sure to master the fine art of making a clean break on the tablet. Also be sure that your doctor understands what you are doing, and the instructions on the medication bottle read accord-ingly. *And never try to halve doses of a capsule by dumping out part of the powder.*

You will also want to check on the medication part of your in-surance plan. You may not have elected to participate in the drug plan in the past, but it's probably a good idea now, if you're going to be filling a prescription for antihypertensive medications every month.

What about combination drugs? If you take at least two antihy-pertensive drugs, your doctor may prescribe them in a combined form. For example, if you take propranolol and hydrochlorothia-zide each day, you may be able to take these in combination in the same tablet. While this is very convenient, and may add to your compliance in taking your medications, it also might cost more than purchasing the medications separately. Bottom line: Combi-nation drugs are sometimes a good idea, but not as a money saver.

Finally, a note of caution. Many people find that medications are less expensive in foreign countries. This is sometimes true. However, buying medications outside the United States or Canada can be risky. Many foreign countries have much lower standards for quality and enforcement of laws relating to quality. Further-more, medications come in different strengths and even have dif-ferent names in other countries. And you can't expect your doc-tor to be able to help you. After all, keeping track of the thousands of medications available in the United States is complicated enough! While you may save some money abroad, there's a good chance it'll be a false economy. Bottom line: If you're an Ameri-can, don't buy medications outside the United States or Canada unless you actually live in another country, and you can rely on your doctor there to get a high-quality medication, for whatever the cost.

Tests

You may be reluctant to undergo certain tests your doctor may want to order, on the basis of cost or any other reason. However, keep in mind that as a "silent" disease, many side effects of the medications, as well as the effects of hypertension itself on target organs, can be detected only by tests. Your best approach is to be certain that you thoroughly understand every test your doctor orders, why it was ordered, and how its result may affect your treatment. Such dialogue is the best insurance that tests will be truly worth the cost, without compromising your doctor's ability to give you the best possible care.

Diet

Although special foods under diet labels can be very convenient, they also can be expensive.

You can control your sodium, fat, and calorie intake without buying such "health foods." A good cookbook, such as *The American Heart Association Cookbook,* tells you how. Furthermore, the new federal food labeling laws make it easy to know exactly how much of the important nutrients are contained in almost all foods. If you need more help, your doctor can recommend a good nutritionist to consult.

If you visit a "health food store," you might also see many products claiming to be good for hypertension—like fish oil, vitamins, and pills containing metals like magnesium, manganese, and chromium. Remember, these places have the right to claim almost anything they want (and they will), without proof to back up their claims. If you need magnesium, your doctor will tell you so. Your local pharmacist is another convenient, reliable source of advice about the efficacy of such nonprescription products.

Doctors

Your visits to the doctor should be a lot less frequent after your blood pressure is stabilized. That's when you need to sit down with your doctor and discuss the "game plan" from then on, which includes the frequency of scheduled office visits, and what is to be done each time.

You should also have a good understanding of what can be handled by telephone. For example, a change in your morning blood pressure reading, or a possible medication side effect, are questions often easily handled by telephone, sometimes immediately by the nurse.

And remember: Pediatricians, family practitioners, internists, and other primary-care physicians are well qualified to treat hypertension. Chances are you will never need to consult a physician specializing in hypertension, usually a nephrologist, but your personal physician will refer you if necessary.

At Home

As we discussed in chapter 5, it is probably a good idea to learn how to take your blood pressure yourself. Keep an accurate daily log of your readings, and some trips to the doctor's office may be eliminated.

Home Sweet Home
Research shows that up to 30% of doctor visits could be eliminated by home BP measurements, at a national savings of $300 million per year.

The Job

Having hypertension should not cause any lost workdays or lost wages, except when a visit to the doctor requires taking time off.

Medications themselves *shouldn't* interfere, either. But if you do find that concentration is more difficult, or if you fatigue easily, or if for any other reason you have trouble at work, you should tell your doctor right away. The medication you're on could be the culprit, even after you've been on it awhile.

Large employers with clinics are excellent places to have your blood pressure checked at no cost. And this is a convenient place to have your own BP monitor checked for accuracy now and then, as well.

It's Your Turn

1. What are you doing that may help reduce your medication requirements to control your BP?

- ❑ Losing weight
- ❑ Reducing salt intake
- ❑ Reducing alcohol intake
- ❑ Exercising regularly

2. Does your health plan cover drug costs?

❑ Yes   ❑ No

If no, you should contact your plan representative to see if a drug plan is available.

3. Are you having any side effects from your BP medications causing you to:

Take any other medications? (list)*

_____

_____

Have additional tests on a regular basis? (list)*

_____

_____

Visit the doctor more often?*

❑ Yes   ❑ No

Miss work or alter you work routine?*

❑ Yes   ❑ No

If yes, how? _____

*Discuss this with your doctor if you haven't already done so or you are unsure of the answer.

7

Special Folks

Children

THE BLOOD PRESSURE normally rises throughout childhood and adolescence, finally reaching a plateau in early adulthood. Then it pretty much stays at that level, unless adult hypertension takes place.

Hypertension is uncommon in children and teenagers, but it does occur, and it can be a very serious problem. Children and adolescents should have their BPs checked yearly, especially if there is a family history of hypertension. Usually, it is on such "routine" exams that hypertension is first detected.

> **That's a Lot of Kids**
> 2.8 million children, ages 6 to 17, have hypertension.

Place Your Bets
If one parent has hypertension, each child has a 25% chance of having hypertension. If both parents have hypertension, the odds rise to 60% for each child.

Diagnosis

Childhood hypertension tends to be "silent." When hypertension causes symptoms in children, the disease is usually severe. Symptoms include headache, tiredness, blurred vision, nosebleeds, and nausea.

In adolescents, the possibility of alcohol, cocaine, and other substance abuse should be kept in mind when the blood pressure is elevated. Anabolic steroids, which are popular among body-building teenagers, especially athletes, should also be considered.

The family history is usually much more revealing, as hypertension and other forms of cardiovascular disease are common in blood relatives. For this reason, both parents, all brothers and sisters, and other close relatives

> **It's in the Genes**
> The BPs of:
> • Parents are closer to natural children than adopted children
> • Identical twins are closer than non-identical twins

of children with hypertension should have their own BPs followed closely.

A child's blood pressure normally swings widely from hour to hour, even more so than an adult's. This has to be taken into account when measuring the blood pressure, and also means that many measurements have to be taken before deciding that a young person truly has hypertension.

But what should the BP be?

The pediatrician uses a chart to determine a child's normal blood pressure. Using the chart, a child does not have hypertension unless:

- The child's average BP is 20mm Hg over the average of 95 percent of children of that age and sex.

- The child's average BP is based on several readings over days, weeks, even months.

Pediatricians Can't Remember All That

The pediatrician uses a chart that tells what the BP should be at any given age. The BP is elevated when it's:

- 96 (systolic) or higher at seven days of age
- 116/76 or higher at three years
- 126/82 or higher at ten years

Just like in adults, once it is decided that hypertension is definitely present, an evaluation is important to determine whether it is the primary or secondary type. However, there is usually more emphasis placed on searching for the presence of other diseases, because secondary hypertension is more common in children than in adults. Secondary hypertension is especially likely if the child is a newborn, or very young, or if the BPs are very high. Kidney abnormalities are often the cause of secondary hypertension.

Finally, when hypertension is diagnosed, the evaluation should include assessment of other risk factors, especially the blood lipids.

Treatment

When secondary hypertension is present, the treatment is focused on correcting the underlying cause. However, the majority of children with hypertension have the primary form, which is managed the same in children as adults, with lifestyle adjustments and medications. These are spelled out in chapters 3 and 4. There are, however, some notable differences, such as very careful attention to avoiding dietary deficiencies (which could harm the child's physical development) and lower drug doses, which are determined by the child's weight. Proper exercise and weight control are just as important as in adults.

Home blood pressure monitoring can be very valuable in helping the doctor prescribe treatment. It is necessary to use smaller cuff sizes for children's small arms, in order to avoid obtaining blood pressures that are falsely low.

Finally, a special note of caution. *Children with hypertension must not be made to feel somehow abnormal or different from other children.* For example, unless severe or uncontrolled hypertension is present, restriction from sports is usually not a good idea, and should be carefully considered with your doctor's guidance before making a final decision. Serious psychological consequences can result from unnecessary interference with a child's normal childhood desires and activities.

Pregnancy

This is a pretty complicated subject, because pregnancy itself is complex. So we're going to give you only some of the highlights of hypertension in pregnancy.

Hypertension can occur in pregnancy in the form of:

- *Chronic (primary or secondary) hypertension,* as we've discussed throughout the book, perhaps uncovered for the first time as a result of repeated visits to the obstetrician.

- *Temporary hypertension,* which disappears after pregnancy is completed.

- *Toxemia of pregnancy,* which occurs in the second and third trimesters and disappears after pregnancy.

- *Chronic hypertension with superimposed toxemia of pregnancy.*

Chronic Hypertension

The vast majority of pregnant women with chronic hypertension do just fine. However, about 15 percent get complications, usually due to *toxemia of pregnancy*. These complications are more likely to occur in women over thirty, and women with long-standing hypertension.

For your and your baby's protection, if you are already being treated for hypertension, *it is crucial that you review your medications and their doses with your physician as soon as you become pregnant, and regularly throughout pregnancy.* You should *not* take ACE inhibitors during pregnancy. Other medications may also carry risks that your doctor will know about.

When hypertension develops during pregnancy, doctors are generally not very aggressive in starting drug therapy. *JNC V* recommends that antihypertensive medication not be started unless the diastolic BP is 100 or greater. The reason for this is the possibility that a medication would reduce the blood flow to the placenta, endangering the baby, with no short-term benefit to the mother when the BP is only mildly elevated.

Toxemia of Pregnancy (TOP)

As we said, pregnancy is a little complicated. For example, the blood pressure normally falls during pregnancy, for reasons your obstetrician can explain if you really want to know. Consequently, what seems like a normal BP may actually be an elevation in pregnancy.

What is toxemia of pregnancy? It is a condition in which the small arteries become narrowed as a result of the artery walls becoming overly sensitive, termed *vasospasm*. The narrowing of the arteries elevates the blood pressure. The cause is unknown. However, as we mentioned, women who have chronic hypertension before they ever become pregnant are especially vulnerable to TOP. It is more common among women with their first pregnancy.

The first evidence of TOP occurs with the phase called *preeclampsia*, which occurs after the twentieth week. Preeclampsia is marked by a rise in the blood pressure, protein in the urine, blood tests showing abnormal kidney function, edema in the legs, blood clotting abnormalities, abnormal liver function tests, and signs of heart failure.

Treatment of preeclampsia requires bed rest and close control of the blood pressure, sometimes requiring hospitalization for careful observation and early induction of labor to prevent progression to eclampsia. Other measures to prevent and treat this condition, such as the use of aspirin, are the subject of a great deal of research.

Preeclampsia can rapidly develop into *eclampsia,* a genuine emergency in which convulsions take place. Symptoms of eclampsia include *headache, changes in vision,* and *abdominal pain.* Both the mother's and her baby's lives are threatened by eclampsia, which is treated as an emergency with special medications followed by induction of labor and delivery of the baby as soon as it's safe to do so.

Fortunately, toxemia of pregnancy usually resolves rapidly following delivery.

Because women who have chronic hypertension have an increased chance of developing toxemia of pregnancy, they should have their BPs closely monitored throughout pregnancy. Close observation is advised if the diastolic BP rises above 75mm Hg in the second trimester, and over 85mm Hg in the third trimester. (Remember, these levels can actually be *elevations,* because the BP normally *falls* during pregnancy.)

Breast-feeding

A final note of caution after pregnancy. Mothers who breast-feed should talk to their doctors about antihypertensive medications (and all other medications, too), because many drugs are secreted in the mother's milk. Diuretics may have to be discontinued because they cause a reduction in milk production.

African-Americans

Hypertension is the most serious health problem among African-Americans in the United States today.

Members of this population, especially men, tend to develop hypertension at a young age, and have a more severe and progressive form of it. As-

More Research Needed

There is little information on hypertension in other races and ethnic groups, including Native Americans, Asians, Pacific Islanders, and Hispanics.

sociated conditions and complications such as stroke, kidney damage, heart attack, heart failure, and even premature death are also more common.

Fortunately, even though hypertension is a particularly serious disease in African-Americans, treatment is very effective in preventing these complications. This begins with the lifestyle changes discussed in chapter 3. Dietary restriction of salt and fats, careful control of weight, and moderation of alcohol intake are all important.

Treatment with antihypertensive medications can be very effective. Diuretics have proven very beneficial in treating hypertension in African-Americans. Calcium blockers, alpha-blockers, and the alpha-beta-blockers are also beneficial. However, beta-blockers and ACE inhibitors may not work as well when given alone.

Seniors

Half of all people over sixty-five have hypertension. This is usually primary hypertension, but a secondary form, often due to blockage of the renal artery by atherosclerosis, should be suspected if hypertension develops quickly in an older person.

We've already addressed the problem of systolic hypertension in chapter 2. This problem is pretty much confined to older ages, and accounts for two-thirds of the cases of hypertension in the elderly.

Contrary to what we believed only a few years ago, research has proven that an elevated systolic pressure demands treatment, even if the diastolic pressure remains normal.

Hypertension in seniors is sometimes falsely diagnosed. This occurs because with age the arteries become stiff, making it difficult for the inflated manometer cuff to compress the arteries when the BP is being taken. As a result, the BP appears to be high, when it actually isn't. This is called *pseudohypertension*, which your doctor has a clever way of discovering. Pure pseudohypertension is not dangerous and doesn't require any form of treatment.

Another precaution about taking the BP: Older folks tend to have even more hour-to-hour fluctuations in their BPs than younger people. For example, their BPs sometimes fall considerably after meals. So *serial* measurements, rather than reliance on a single reading, can be very important.

Our Clever Doctors

Faced with the question of pseudohypertension, doctors employ an old trick first used by an idol of theirs, the great Sir William Osler, to uncover the truth. Using "Osler's Maneuver," they pump up the manometer cuff above the suspicious systolic pressure, then palpate the radial artery (down at the wrist). If they feel a pulsation, the brachial artery is assumed calcified, and the BP isn't as high as the manometer says.

When hypertension is first diagnosed, unless it is very high, lifestyle changes should be tried for a few months, because these can be very effective. Exercise, salt restriction, reduction of alcohol intake, and weight loss can help a lot, but must be carried out under the doctor's close guidance. There should be special attention paid to any other medications that may be elevating the blood pressure. This is particularly true for the NSAIDs, which are commonly taken for arthritis and other aches and pains in older folks.

Drug treatment of hypertension in the elderly has proven to be very worthwhile, in terms of preventing complications. However, this should be done very cautiously, to avoid dropping the BP too much, especially in the upright position *(postural hypotension)*, which was discussed in chapter 5. Sudden falls leading to hip fractures can result. Therefore, BP readings in seniors should include measurements *both sitting and standing*.

Another reason for *carefully* lowering the BP in this age group is the so-called J-curve theory, which reasons that it is possible to lower the BP so much that vital organs, especially the heart, may have their blood flow reduced. This is also discussed in chapter 4.

Doses of medications are usually started lower, and increased more slowly, in the elderly. This is because the elderly are more susceptible to side effects with medications. Particular care should be taken with diuretics, which can cause dehydration, wash too much potassium out of the body, and elevate the uric acid (causing gout) and blood sugar.

Many older women take estrogen and other hormones to replace those hormones lost after menopause. Hypertension is *usu-*

ally not a contraindication to modern postmenopausal hormone replacement therapy (HRT), but some of the older medications containing large amounts of estrogen can raise the BP significantly. Be sure to talk with your doctor about the right dose of HRT. And be certain to have your BP checked regularly if you take HRT.

Diabetes Mellitus

There are many links between diabetes mellitus and hypertension. The reason isn't known for certain, but many theories center on the role of insulin resistance in the body's metabolism and control of blood pressure.

For whatever the reason, diabetes and hypertension share many of the same cardiovascular complications, especially heart attack and stroke. And obesity and abnormal blood fats are common in both.

Therefore the control of risk factors in people with diabetes mellitus often includes treatment of hypertension. *JNC V* recommends that the blood pressure be maintained at 130/85 or less in diabetics.

Diabetics can take the same medications as we've described in chapter 4, with some special precautions:

- If a *diuretic* is taken, it is important to maintain a normal potassium level, because low potassium may elevate the blood sugar. The blood sugar, blood level fats, and uric acid all need to be watched carefully.

- *Beta-blockers* can worsen the blood sugar, and can "mask" the symptoms of low blood sugar as well as interfere with the way that the body naturally corrects low blood sugar when it does occur.

- *Alpha-1 blockers* can worsen orthostatic hypotension, which diabetics are prone to develop.

- *ACE inhibitors* can elevate the potassium.

It's Your Turn

1. If your child has hypertension:
   Have you, the child's other parent, and the child's brothers and sisters all had their BPs checked?
   ❑ Yes   ❑ No*

   Has your child's cholesterol been checked?
   ❑ Yes   ❑ No*
   If yes, state value: _____

2. If you are pregnant, what is your average BP?*
   First trimester _____
   Second trimester _____
   Third trimester _____

3. If you are African-American, have any of the following been effective in lowering your BP?
   ❑ Reducing salt intake*
   ❑ Reducing alcohol intake*
   ❑ Weight loss*

4. If you are a senior citizen:
   Are you being actively treated for your BP, even if only the systolic pressure is significantly elevated?
   ❑ Yes   ❑ No*

   Do you ever get light-headed when arising from reclining or sitting?
   ❑ Yes*   ❑ No

   Do you measure your BP both sitting and standing?
   ❑ Yes   ❑ No*

5. If you have diabetes mellitus and are on antihypertensive medication:

Do you know your potassium level?

❑ Yes   ❑ No*

6. Has any aspect of your control of diabetes worsened since you have been on antihypertensive medications?

❑ Yes*   ❑ No

If yes, state what: _____

7. For everyone: Do you (or does your child) smoke cigarettes or use any other form of tobacco?

❑ Yes   ❑ No

If "yes," QUIT!

*Discuss this with your doctor if you haven't already done so or if you are unsure of the answer.

8

Myths and Realities: Commonly Asked Questions

ONLY WEATHER bulletins grab people's attention faster than health news on television. Which makes perfect sense. What can be more important to our very lives (other than an approaching tornado) than what's going on in health care?

So, thanks to the most advanced and prolific communications system in the world, Americans are very well versed on our ailments and how they are treated. The problem is, not all that we see, read, or hear is correct. And things we once believed to be true, but subsequently learned to be false, often don't get back to us.

That's why we thought this section would be a good idea. By the way, if you have read some of these things before in this book, it's because we believe that a little repetition is a good thing.

What is an elevated blood pressure?

An elevated blood pressure is a systolic pressure of 140 or higher, or a diastolic pressure of 90 or higher.

How many people have high blood pressure?

It's estimated that about sixty-four million people have high blood pressure in the United States. Some surveys show that less than half of these people may know it.

At what age does hypertension usually start?

Most people are over age thirty-five when hypertension is first detected. However, the initial diagnosis can occur at any time, from birth through very old age.

Does hypertension come and go?

No. Once hypertension is established, it's always there. Regardless how good you feel, or how well medications control the blood pressure, hypertension does not go away.

Is there any cure for hypertension?

Primary hypertension can be controlled but not cured. Some instances of secondary hypertension, which affects 10 percent or less of people with hypertension, can be cured with surgery.

If you have hypertension, will your children get hypertension too?

If one parent has hypertension, each child has a 25 percent chance of developing hypertension as well. If both parents have hypertension, the odds rise to 60 percent.

Do many children have high blood pressure?

It's estimated that 2.8 million children ages six to seventeen have high blood pressure. So hypertension is neither common nor rare in children.

Does stress cause hypertension?

No. Stress can raise the blood pressure temporarily, but it does not cause the disease we call hypertension. Some people are more "sensitive" to blood pressure elevations caused by stress.

What happens if you don't control your blood pressure?

Hypertension markedly increases the risk for heart attack, strokes, heart failure, kidney failure, and blockages and aneurysms of the arteries.

Is treating hypertension really beneficial?

Yes. Studies show that people who are effectively treated for hypertension suffer less from diseases of the heart and blood vessels than those who are not treated.

Is it important to measure your own blood pressure?

Yes. Measuring your blood pressure at home gives your doctor a much better indication of how well your treatment is working at times other than while you are in the office. This can also reduce the number of visits to the doctor's office after your "goal" blood pressure is reached, saving time and expense.

Which is the best home blood pressure measuring device?

The aneroid type is inexpensive and reliable, as long as it is kept calibrated. Automated devices are expensive and tend to be less accurate. Mercury manometers are the most accurate, but are expensive and bulky. Before purchasing your own manometer, do a little research, including talking to your doctor and pharmacist.

What foods should you eat if you have hypertension?

In general you want to eat foods that are low in fat and sodium, with adequate amounts of potassium and calcium in your daily diet. This means more emphasis on fruits and vegetables, and less consumption of processed foods and animal products, especially those high in fat and sodium. (Read labels carefully.)

Is it important to watch your weight?

Absolutely. Know what your weight should be, get it down to that level, and keep it there. This alone can have a marked effect on your blood pressure.

Why a low-sodium diet?

Too much sodium elevates many people's blood pressure. The average American consumes about *twenty-four times* what the body needs.

How do we get so much sodium?

The most obvious source is ordinary table salt. But there are plenty of other common sodium-containing products: MSG (monosodium glutamate), baking soda, baking powder, and commercially prepared foods, such as frozen dinners and canned foods.

What about salt substitutes?

If you must "salt," try a low-sodium salt substitute (there are lots out there, in the form of potassium salts). Better yet, try other seasonings to enhance flavor, such as allspice, almond extract, basil, bay leaves, caraway seeds, chives, curry, dill, and vinegar. Experiment with new tastes!

What about fat in the diet?

Dietary fats elevate the cholesterol, which is another powerful risk factor for atherosclerosis. Along with sodium, fats should be restricted—how much depends on the cholesterol level in the blood stream.

What about eating more calcium to lower blood pressure?

Some studies have shown that consuming more calcium helps lower blood pressure a little, but not enough to be a treatment for hypertension. However, it is a good idea to eat calcium-rich foods for other reasons, especially for its protection against osteoporosis.

What about exercise?

The right exercise can be an important part of controlling your blood pressure (and other risk factors, like weight). If you're already exercising regularly, you should continue, *as long as your doctor approves.* Before beginning any new exercise program, you should also discuss it with your doctor.

What is the best kind of exercise to help lower blood pressure?

Exercise that increases your heartbeat for an extended period of time is best. Excellent activities include walking, swimming, cross-country skiing, and bicycling, and all can be done without special equipment. If those sorts of activities are too strenuous for you, even modest activity like gardening can be beneficial. Stay away from isometric forms of exercise, such as weight lifting.

What about exercise and medications?

Some blood pressure medications prevent the normal changes your body must undergo for exercise. As a result, you could have difficulties during or after exercise, such as tiring easily, feeling light-headed, or even passing out. Many doctors insist on an exercise test prior to beginning, or even continuing, an exercise program for this reason. *Make sure to check with your doctor to see if it's safe to exercise.*

Is biofeedback therapy an alternative to antihypertensive medications?

No. There is no evidence that this is an effective treatment of hypertension.

Should people with hypertension take tranquilizers?

Not to treat the hypertension. The indications for administering sedatives, for daytime use or for sleep, are no different for people with hypertension than they are for anyone else.

Can you ever discontinue your medications?

Seldom. And then only after you have been well controlled for a while, and *only under your doctor's orders.* Even if that works, you must continue to monitor your blood pressure and keep following good lifestyle practices, especially weight control.

What if you can't afford the medications or other treatment?

Make sure you have a drug plan, if it's available. Be sure to fully use all the benefits you *need* under your personal health insurance, Medicare, state programs, and organizations such as NARP. A number of other organizations offer help with insurance questions and similar problems: Visiting Nurse Association, Adult Activity Centers, social service agencies, and public health departments.

What about oral contraceptives?

All estrogen-containing drugs can elevate the blood pressure. Therefore, if you have hypertension and take oral contraceptives, talk to your doctor. You may need another form of birth control.

What about alcohol and hypertension? Do you have to stop drinking?

Alcohol elevates the blood pressure. Therefore you need to abstain or limit your intake to moderate levels, which is about one ounce or less of ethanol a day, or twenty-four ounces of beer, eight ounces of wine, or two ounces of one hundred-proof whiskey.

What about pregnancy and hypertension?

Eighty-five percent of pregnant women with hypertension have normal pregnancies. However, failure to control high blood pressure during pregnancy increases the risk for developing toxemia of pregnancy and fetal complications.

Do medications affect fetal development?

Some drugs have been used for many years without any apparent danger to the fetus and can be used without risk during pregnancy. However, new studies come out regularly and you should talk about any medications with your doctor if you are pregnant. One type of drug that *definitely should not* be taken during pregnancy is an ACE inhibitor, because it can harm the unborn baby.

*What about nursing your baby if you take
antihypertensive medication?*

Almost every medicine enters breast milk, some in much
higher concentrations than others. Therefore it is very
important to talk to your doctor about the safety of nursing if you are on an antihypertensive medication, or any
other drug.

*Are members of certain ethnic groups more likely
to become hypertensive?*

Yes. This is the most serious health problem in African-
Americans. We're not sure about other ethnic groups.

*My grandmother is eighty and has hypertension.
Is she too old to be taking a drug for her blood pressure?*

You are never too old to try to prevent a stroke or a heart
attack. Antihypertensive medications are effective in the
elderly.

9

A Final Thought

BY NOW YOU should be well on your way toward a solid understanding of hypertension, especially how high blood pressure relates to you personally and what you can do about it.

So this is a good time to think about the future.

Maybe the best way to get an idea about tomorrow is to look at yesterday. If we know the direction we've come from, we can get a good idea where we're going.

The Veterans Cooperative Study, which was the first proof that treating hypertension could prevent cardiovascular disease, was completed less than thirty years ago. Look what's happened since:

- Beta-blockers, calcium antagonists, and ACE inhibitors have all come into use, virtually revolutionizing drug treatment.

- The incidence of coronary heart disease has fallen dramatically.

- The incidence of stroke has fallen even more.

- New medications to prevent acute blood-vessel blockage have been developed, and it's been discovered that good old aspirin helps to prevent blood clots.

- We've gained new insight into blood lipids, such as the presence of a "protective" form of cholesterol—the HDL cholesterol.

- Powerful new drugs to lower the cholesterol have become available.

• Evidence that we can actually prevent damage to the heart muscle and kidneys with medications is rapidly emerging.

• And the list goes on. . . .

In short, if the recent past is any indication, our ability to manage hypertension and prevent its complications will only improve—probably by a lot—over the next few years.

Beyond medications, there is exciting new research that will inevitably lead to breakthroughs in underlying causes of hypertension, particularly with respect to genetics. So it's possible that our children might be entirely spared the problem of hypertension, by altering genetic codes that lead to elevated blood pressure. The same is true for other cardiovascular and metabolic problems such as coronary heart disease, lipid abnormalities, and diabetes mellitus.

Who knows, maybe some mad scientist will even figure out the gene that makes us gain weight—and end dieting forever!

But let's not get carried away. You, with help from your doctor, still have to take care of today. We've tried to assist, by telling you some of the details about hypertension that we know can make a difference. Hopefully we've succeeded, at least a little.

Regardless of what we or anyone else says or does, hypertension is still *your* journey to make. And you know, we're confident you are going to make that trip just fine.

Index

(Page numbers in *italic* refer to sidebar information)

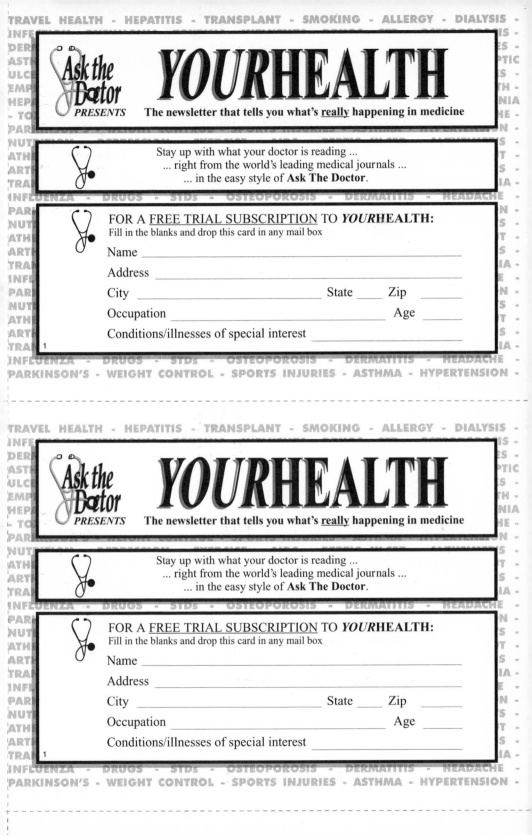

Ask the Doctor *PRESENTS*

*YOUR*HEALTH

The newsletter that tells you what's <u>really</u> happening in medicine

Stay up with what your doctor is reading ...
... right from the world's leading medical journals ...
... in the easy style of **Ask The Doctor**.

FOR A <u>FREE TRIAL SUBSCRIPTION</u> TO *YOUR*HEALTH:
Fill in the blanks and drop this card in any mail box

Name _____

Address _____

City _____ State _____ Zip _____

Occupation _____ Age _____

Conditions/illnesses of special interest _____

1

Ask the Doctor *PRESENTS*

*YOUR*HEALTH

The newsletter that tells you what's <u>really</u> happening in medicine

Stay up with what your doctor is reading ...
... right from the world's leading medical journals ...
... in the easy style of **Ask The Doctor**.

FOR A <u>FREE TRIAL SUBSCRIPTION</u> TO *YOUR*HEALTH:
Fill in the blanks and drop this card in any mail box

Name _____

Address _____

City _____ State _____ Zip _____

Occupation _____ Age _____

Conditions/illnesses of special interest _____

1

BUSINESS REPLY MAIL

FIRST-CLASS PERMIT NO. 364 THE WOODLANDS, TX

POSTAGE WILL BE PAID BY ADDRESSEE

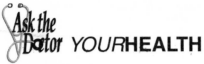 *Ask the* *Doctor* YOUR**HEALTH**

P.O. Box 7725
The Woodlands, Texas 77387-9919

BUSINESS REPLY MAIL

FIRST-CLASS PERMIT NO. 364 THE WOODLANDS, TX

POSTAGE WILL BE PAID BY ADDRESSEE

Ask the *Doctor* YOUR**HEALTH**

P.O. Box 7725
The Woodlands, Texas 77387-9919